Alternative Therapy Sequel: 5

A Treatise on Electro Homoeopathic Pharmacy

By

Prof. Dr. Debasish Kundu

M.D.H., F.F.Hom, F.I.H.M.S., Ph.D.(U.S.A.), D.Sc.(Colombo)

Compiled by

Dr. Ajit Singh

M.Sc.,B.E.M.S., D.A.M., M.F.Hom, D.Acu, D.Litt

Originals

Delhi

1st Edition 2001
2nd Revised & Enlarged Edition 2005
Third Edition 2017

ISBN 13: 978-81-8454-169-4
ISBN 10: 81-8454-169-4

Published By
Originals
A-6, Second Floor, Nimri Commercial Centre,
Ashok Vihar Phase-4, Delhi - 110 052 (India)
Tel.: +91 11 2730 2453 Fax: 011 4706 1936
website: www.Lppindia.com
e-mail: info@Lppindia.com

Printed At
D K Fine Art Press P Ltd.
Delhi-110052

PRINTED IN INDIA

Prof. Dr. Debasish Kundu

M.D.H., F.F.Hom, F.I.H.M.S., Ph.D.(U.S.A.), D.Sc.(Colombo)

Fellow of International Holistic Medical Society, CA, U.S.A.

Fellow of Foundation of Homeopathy, MO, U.S.A.

Fellow of World E.Homeopathy System of Medical Council, Hong Kong

Faculty, International Holistic Medical Society, CA, U.S.A.

Faculty, Association of Independent Natural Science Schools Colleges, Professions & Arts, MO, U.S.A.

Vice-President, American Nutritional Medical Association, CA, U.S.A.

Foreign Bureau Chief (India), Holistic Medical Hylite International, CA, U.S.A.

Visiting Professor, Khulna Homeopathic Medical College & Hospital, Khulna, Bangladesh

Ex-Director General, Mooreland University, U.S.A.

Former Adjunct. Faculty & Associate Professor, Department of Human Behavior, Newport University, U.S.A.

Editor In Chief, International Journal of Homeopathy & Natural Medicines, USA

Editor in Chief, The Internet Journal of Herbal and Plant Medicine, USA

Author,

Diseases of Women,

Natural Medicines,

A Clinical Treatise on Cancer,

Aids & Homeopathy,

Pharmacodynamics,

Aids & Your Sex Life,

Aids & Homeopathy,

Essentials of Acupuncture,

Materia Medica for the New Age Man, etc.

Recipient, Royal Assyrian Order of Merit (OIUCM, 1993)

Laureate, United Nations Dag Hammarskjold Award for Medicine (1995)

Recipient, Special Achievement Award, International Conference on E. Omeopatia, Poretta Terme, Bologna, Italy (2008)

Dr. Ajit Singh

Managing Director, Biome Spagyrics, Jalandhar (Pb).

Secretary, All India Research & Development Organisation of Electrohomeopathy, New Delhi

DEDICATED

To

All Truth Seekers of
Electrohomoeopathy

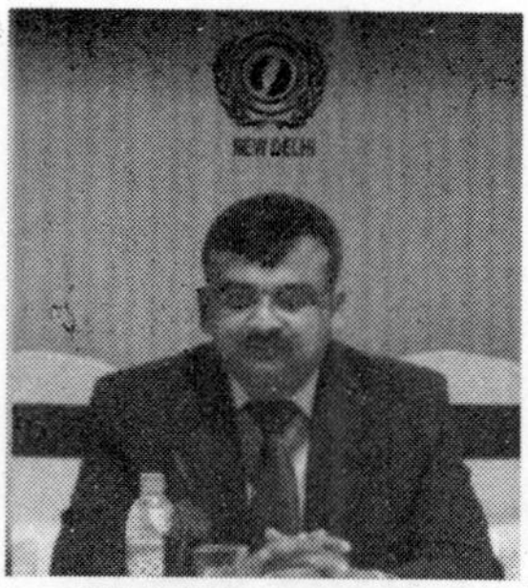

Foreword

I am pleased to have the opportunity to write foreword for the book of Treatise on Electro Homoeopathic Pharmacy which is written by Dr. Debasish Kundu for ADEH students. Because I have a dream for all my Electro Homoeopathic practitioners that one day they must get an official Certificate from any Government Agency and I am happy to say that Maharashtra is the First State in India to offer an Official Electro Homoeopathy Certificate which is being awarded by the Government Agency. Also I have some friends who helped me to fulfill my dream to introduce a Government recognised ADVANCE DIPLOMA IN ELECTRO HOMOEOPATHY (ADEH) course in Maharashtra.

When word comes "ADVANCED" means something new and scientific, so while reading the contents of the book, I found something new and advanced. Since long time Dr. Kundu is writing books on different subjects which are very easy to understand and rich in contents, so I believe this book will help all the Students, Practitioners & Lovers of Electro-Homoeopathy besides students in perusing ADEH examination which contains the study material mentioned in Syllabus by MSBVE, Mumbai. This entire course material will help to improve the knowledge in Electro Homoeopathy subject.

Dr. Trideep Guha
BPTH, MD (ECH) MBA, Ph.D., MRCE (USA)
Chairman
Educational & Medical/Paramedical Council of India
Executive Member:
Paramedical Syllabus Committee,
MSBVEE, Mumbai (Govt. of Maharashtra)

Email id
drtrideep.g@gmail.com, empci@hotmail.com
Visit us at :
www.empci.com

Published By

Originals

A-6, Second Floor, Nimri Commercial Centre,
Ashok Vihar Phase-4, Delhi - 110 052 (India)
Tel.: +91 11 2730 2453 Fax: 011 4706 1936
Website: www.Lppindia.com
e-mail: info@Lppindia.com

In Association with

ADEH PRACTISIONERS ASSOCIATION MAHARASHTRA
N-123, Second floor, Infront of Devanjali flats,
Reshimbag, City & District : Nagpur
State : Maharashtra Country : INDIA
Phone : +91-712-2700606, +91-712-2700651, +91-712-2700777

Foreword

Dr. Debasish Kundu in this work "Pharmacopedics in Electro-Homoeopathy", has summarized in details the central core of the art of preparation of Electro-Homoeopathic Remedies. One think should be clearified, and it is that the original E.H. remedies formulas are not knew at the moment in their entire contenents and method of preparation. Indeed this has been also declared by the Mattei's Count Family, living today. The original laboratories of Mattei's Family has been closed more than thirthy years ago.

However, the research conducted by Dr. Debasish Kundu, Dr. Ajit Singh and other researchers in this field, In India, Europe and America mainly, are to be taken in big considerations. I believe that Dr. Kundu here has centered the main argument of E.H.: whatever the ingredients, the remedies has to be prepared by an alchemic-spagyric method. The formulas of E.H. as we know, has been mainly reported by German pharmacists and researcher, in contact with Count Cesare Mattei, and published after the Count Mattei's death (1896), about at the time of first years of 1900. From that ingredients and method of preparation, we have basically the actual method of production. Obviously, any system to improve it should to be accepted.

The efford to reach a good, natural, safe E.H. medicines is a remarkable work, in which Dr. Kundu and others are dedicating generously, from many years, their lives.

Dr. Fabio Ambrosi
Director,
Universita Internazionale Della Nouva Medicina, Milan,
Deptt.Natural Medicines, Italy, Oderzo-Venice,
1st July 2005

American Nutritional Medical Association

P.O.Box 66005 Stockton,CA 95206 U.S.A.
Tel: (209) 464-3884, Fax: (209) 464-2943,
E-Mail: anmainc@sify.com

President
Prof. Malik A.K. Awan, Ph.D
Stockton, California, U.S.A.
E-Mail: drawan10@aol.com

Vice President
Dr. Adrian O. Starchild, M.D.
Lake Arenal, Costa Rica
E-Mail:institutebiomed@san.rr.com

Foreword

It gives me a great pleasure to foreword the book "A treatise on Electrohomoeopathic Pharmacy" by Dr. Debasish Kundu and Dr.Ajit Singh. I may recall that myself with Dr. Starchild visited the Mattei Castle in Bologna in 2000 and an agreement was made offer ing Dr.Starchild to take internal and external filiming and photos of the La Rochetta Castle built by Count Mattei. The current owners the Stefanelli's agreed to see Dr. Starchild in January 2002 and take photos inside the historic monument (the first since Stefanelli's became owners of the castle, they had even turned down professors from Bologna and Fircnze from doing so), what Dr. Starchild find out when arrived, the original Electrohomoeopathy fermenting chamber, books and everything relating to Electro-homoeopathy had been either misplaced or destroyed on the passing of the Heir of the Count of when the Stefanelli's purchased the property. The castle is now nothing more than a piece of history. To be frank there is currently no manufacturer of the cohobated spagyric remedies prepared according to secrets so closely held by Count Mattei. However one last remaining source, there was one student who Count Mattei shared his valuable secrets with , besides his mysterious heir and adopted son Signor Ventrouli Mattei, and that was one German Scientist Theodore Krauss who resided briefly with the Count to spread the knowledge of Electrohomoeopathy in Germany, he translated neumerous texts from Italian to German and opened the ISO-Arznemittel in Regensburg, Germany, on the eastern side of Bavaria and even taught Russian homeopaths the art of Electrohomoeopathy, which back in early 1920's flourished in Russia. Since the passing of Dr. Krauss the company struggled to remain in Regensburg, and new hands exchanges different ideas on what company should produce then they produce homeopathic and naturopathic medicines and in the later part of 1990's even produced Cosmetics. They eventually sold out in the 1990's to one of the leading allopathic firms in Germany and moved to Karlsruhe, and have abandoned the involvement of Electrohomoeopathy. Dr. Starchild visited their manufacturing facilities in 1994 and found that the remedies are produced in accordance to Krauss method, but the principles of Electrohomoeopathy coincided with the teachings and philosophy of Count Mattei in which the remedies are extracted through Alchemical principles by separating and re-uniting Salt, Sulphur and Mercury.

I personally feel that the method discussed here is the lost Mattei method of extracting cohobated remedies, the true Spagyrica!

Prof. Dr. Sir Malik A.K. Awan
B.S.,M.S. (Psychology), Ph.D. (London)
President & CE

MANAV SEWA PARMO DHARAM

Electrohomoeopathic Doctors Association

Punjab (Regd. No. 119/2000)

Foreword

As per Electrohomoeopathy Disease is the result of Vitiation of Blood and Lymph and in language of Biochemistry this condition is simply a deficiency of minerals and trace elements. To fill up this deficiency Mattei prepared his medicines by process of Spagyric Cohobation, these Spagyric medicines are rich in minerals properties and thus able to fulfill the requirements of the living organisms to regain the health. By intake of Electrohomoeopathic remedies all parts of our body are energised and thus help to eradicate or ward off any kind of communicable diseases.

The Electrohomoeopathy is a classic system of medicine of Europe but it has now spread all over the world. Its medicines not only cure but brings a sence of well-being.

The Authors have written the scattered art of Electrohomoeopathy Pharmacy in very easy and understandable language.

I am hopeful that the formidable efforts undertaken by the Authors would achieve the target of fulfilling the need of a standard text on Electrohomoeopathy pharmacy.

Dr. Tarsem Singh,
MDEH (Gold Medalist), D.Sc.(Hon. Causa) General Secretary

Excerpts From Foreword by Some Eminent Personalities

(1)

I have read the book 'A Treatise on Electro Homeopathic Pharmacy' written by Dr. Debasish Kundu and Dr. Ajit Singh it is in one word breakthrough in Electro Homeopathy. I think this book will serve the long awaited need of a text on Electro Homeopathy Pharmacy, I must congratulate the authors for their unique work.

Dr. B. B. Upreti Ph.D.
General Secretary, All Nepal Electro Homeopathic Medical Association, Kathmandu, Nepal

(2)

'A Treatise on Electro Homeopathic Pharmacy' is an excellent introduction to the system of Electro Homeopathic Pharmacy and one that is concise, direct, and easy to understand , it covers all the main concepts, techniques and deliberations in a way that is both interesting and informative, in perfect harmony of it's scientific aspects and traditions. The book provides Electro Homeopathic Secrets for health and well being for every citizen of the earth.

Dr. Incesstio Terro Ph.D.
Electro Homeopathic Scientist & Director, International Holistic Medical Society, Spain Chapter

(3)

This book is a pioneering effort in the history of Electro-homoeopathy. I am sure this will stimulate the Unexplored era of this Unique healing art of Electrohomoeopathy. The Authors have discussed the Pharmaceutical system extensively and collectively. The journey can be exciting enough for the truth seekers.

Prof. Dr. Mohd. Hanif Ph.D
President, Al-Shifa Institute for Complementary Medicines,
Lahore, Pakistan.

(4)

I have gone through the book entitled "A treatise on Electrohomoeopathic Pharmacy". The methods described by the Authors attracted me at the glance and I wanted to ascertain the facts by direct experimentation. Hence I followed their method and found accurate. I have not even the slightest doubt about the success of Electrohomoeopathy in the medical world.

Prof. Dr. Chowdhury Mahabubul Haque, Ph.D
Principal,
Chowdhury Homoeopathic and Paramedical College,
Daulatpur, Khulna, Bangladesh.

(5)

I have the privilege to personally know the authors as outstanding physicians in the field of Electrohomoeopathy. Their thrilling new book "A treatise on Electrohomoeopathic Pharmacy" seems to have revolutionized the Electrohomoeopathy medical science. I believe the authors will continue to prove a boon to the ailing Humanity.

Dr. D. Singh BEMS, MD (AM)
Director, Sweden Medical Council of Electrohomoeopathy,
Norsborg, Sweden

(6)

Drs. Kundu and Singh , the authors of the book "A Treatise on Electro Homeopathic Pharmacy" are renowned Electrohomoeopaths and are credited with having cured many so called incurable cases. They now have rediscovered a new technique for achieving the classic Mattei remedies. In this approach of the authors there is scientific representation of electrohomoeopathic pharmacy as the findings and results are statistically analyzed. The mysteries of nature can only be revealed by scientific experimentations. The authors enthusiasm for scientific investigations has compelled me these few lines in appreciations. I wish them a great success in their endeavors.

Dr. Sukhninder Singh MD(EH) Director, Mattei Board of Electrohomoeopathy, Coventry, U.K.

(7)

I am quite impressed seeing the depthness of the unique work done by the authors. They have represented the Electrohomoeopathy Pharmacy in its true shape and quite acceptable format. The matter discussed in the book is worth reading. It could be debated whether Electrohomoeopathy is to be called the Perfected or Spagyric Homoeopathy. The Zeal of the authors is contagious.

Dr. Harminder Singh Dalla, MSc.
Secretary CBMA, CANADA

Preface to the Third Edition

The contents of this book constitute the evolving field of Electro Homeopathy Pharmacy. One could easily write entire volumes about the topics of each of the chapters in this text, but the task of the authors here was to assimilate this large body of information on Electro Homeopathy Pharmacy and condense it into a useful textbook of manageable size. Each chapter represents a careful distillation of current science, key concepts, and treatments of the subject at hand into an accessible format. For those readers seeking to expand their horizons further, the authors have prepared extensive lists of references at the end of the book to provide the reader with further details.

This third edition discusses the fundamental dimensions of Electro Homeopathy Pharmacy, the various aspects, and the methods employed in its management, with special emphasis on the use of laboratory pharmacy.

We welcome comments, suggestions, and constructive criticism from all our readers.

Dr. Debasish Kundu
Dr. Ajit Singh

Preface

Pharmaceutical procedures form an integral part of our Materia Medica and even the knowledge of Materia Medica remains incomplete if it be not supplemented with the scientific study of pharmaceutical arts and sciences.

The preparation of spagyric remedies is an ancient art. Concurrently, it is a timeless art because the basic principles, which align themselves to the phenomenology and natural laws of space and time, never lose their validity. In the future, the importance of spagyric remedies will increase even further because their potency and effectiveness as a holistic medicine will not only be intuitively realised, but will be also be proven in the same way that the interconnectedness of all life forms on the earth and in the cosmos is now being understood and proven.

The spagyric art of producing a high quality medication is a method in which the transmutation patterns of plants, mineral and metallic substances that normally take place in nature as part of a larger evolutionary cycle, instead take place within a small laboratory setting, where they are quickened through the process of catalysis.

The word spagyric comes from the Greek words spao, which means separate, and ageiro, which means unify. A fundamental law of nature is that of polarity. This can be seen, for example, in the process of breathing: during inhalation, a part separates from the whole, and during exhalation the part again returns to the whole. There is an everchanging process of "dying and becoming", which, however, contains the dynamics of perfection.

The separation and unification processes used in the production of spagyric remedies should be seen as an attempt to increase the life energy found within a plant or mineral. This process of cohobation (elevation) is achieved through repeated distillations in which the distillate is repeatedly reunified with the residue, and the distillation is carried out anew.

Through continual changes in the aggregate conditions of the distillate and through the reunification with the residue in the distillation container, the distillate attains a high level of purity and, at the same time, its effectiveness is dynamised. Certain plants, minerals and metals each have their own specific distillation rhythm, and these are strictly observed. Depending upon the composition and/or structure of the particular mineral or plant needing to be "unlocked", either rhythmic distillations, also called rotations, or circulations, in which the distillations are carried out continually and repeatedly at constant temperature up to 33 times, are used.

The processes of solve and coagula that transpire during laboratory distillation not only refer to the separation and reunification of the distillate and the residue, but primarily refer to the separation of the plant, metal or mineral into the three active principles Mercury, Sulphur and Salt.

Mercury is the transpersonal spirit/mind principle. In a remedy, it is the carrier of information. It is the water element which carries the essence or aroma of the plant.

Sulphur is the soul principle. In a remedy, it represents the "personal" inner qualities and active ingredients within the substance. In plants, it is the fire element and the soul principal of the plant.

Salt is the physical principle. In a remedy,it includes the active ingredients that can be analysed, measured, weighed and even synthesized. In plants it is the earth elements and plant ashes.

It should be clear that sulphur and mercury principles aren't found in synthetically produced remedies. In these types of remedies, only the physical level can be reproduced.

In homeopathy, the mercury principle is attained through the process of potentiation. In this case, it is the information within the substance that has been dynamised.

Spagyric production methods are holistic in every sense of the word. Because of this, their application has nothing to do with suppression, substitution or with the physiological emulation of disturbed life processes, as is the case for synthesized or standardized remedies. In spagyric remedies, information for both the repair and the reorganisation of disturbed regulatory systems are given simultaneously. The most important thing, however, is that the remedy supplies the patient with the life energy that he is lacking so that he can dynamically apply this core information and use regenerating building blocks toward an appropriate repair and re-synthesis.

In addition to this holistic therapy principle in spagyric medicine, the composition of the finished remedies, which are always mixtures, are composed of ingredients that are related to each other through function and or affinity to a particular organ.

For example, there is a holistic remedy specific to the liver and a composition that stimulates the eliminating function specific to the kidneys. These remedies are holistic in the sense that they act on all three levels of the human being and address his relationship to the surrounding cosmos.

In order to produce such a high quality remedy, one naturally also needs high quality starting materials.

All of the plants are dried on silk screens, and it is here, with these plants, that the beginning steps in spagyric production process take place. After observing the care and purity in which these spagyric remedies are prepared within our "toxic" world. Most diseases are the result of a loss of one's own inner biorhythm. People have forgotten that they are a microcosm within a macrocosm and that they are also affected by the natural cosmic and planetary rhythm. Indeed, we can only be healthy and whole when we are coherently attune to these rhythms.

Our immune systems as well as our metabolic processes are dependent upon rhythmic regulation. Every living system is in a rhythmic, vibrating state of balance. Health is a dynamic balance between chaos and order. Disease occurs there where the active rhythm between the poles has been lost. For this reason, a challenge for our day and age is to fundamentally turn away from the dead end street we are on, and to once again search for the true middle way.

The sun and moon, the two representatives of the polar rhythm of our being, complement one another in a harmonious way–there can be no yin without yang, and no yang without yin. It is a gift to have remedies that contain within them the secret of the balance of energies and the structures that they form.

The book 'A Treatise on Electro Homoeopathic Pharmacy' is the result of our years of continuous research and development on the healing art of Electro Homoeopathy, we trust that the fraternity will be benefited with the work, and it should fulfill the need of a standard text on the subject for the professionals and laymen alike.

We are indebted to Dr. Fabio.R. Ambrosi (Italy), Countess Gianna Fadda Mattei (The living Successor of Count Mattei), Alessandro Rapirrini (Italy), Mr. Claudio Carelli (Italy), Dr. Fransceso (Italy), Dr. Incestio Teero, (Spain), Dr.Adrian Oliver Starchild, (Costa Rica), Dr. Axel Helmstadter, (Germany) Prof. Dr. Malik Awan, (USA), Dr. Nic D.Mainferme (U.S.A.), Dr. Ms. Katalin Soltesz, (Hungary), Dr. Rahbeer Kaleemi, (Pakistan), Late Prof. Dr.Anton Jayasuriya (Sri Lanka), Dr. A.

Meera (Sri Lanka), Dr. SyedAbu Sayeed (Bangladesh), Dr. Kamal Chitrakar (Nepal), Dr. H.T. Chan Wah (Malaysia), Dr. Mohd. Zubeir (Mukkah, K.S.A), Dr. Sc.Agr. Claus Geiselhart (ISO-Arzneimittel GmbH & Co. KG,Germany), Mr. Ann Williams (U.K), Dr. Sukhninder Singh (U.K), Mr. Juergen Christian Bauer (Germany), Mr. Uwe Zind (ISO-Arzneimittel GmbH & Co. KG Germany), Dr. Krishma (Sweden), Ms. Elizabeth Ihrig (Bakken Library, USA), Dr. Linda Lanchester (USA), Late Dr. Gurkirpal Singh Bains (U.K), Dr. B.S.Tayagi, Dr. Rajinder Nangal, Dr. Tarsem Singh, Dr. D.K. Pal, Dr. B. Daksh, Dr. Sanjeev Sharma, Dr. Swapan Kr. Chatterjee (Developer of Polydynamics Software), Dr. Uday Bodhankar, Dr. E.Jagan, Dr.P.R. Prathap Singh, Dr. N. N. Misal, Dr. K.C.Mahapatra, Dr. Bharati, Dr. S. Nagendran, Dr. Surinder Singh, Advocate Rajinderr Singh Bains, Dr. Sanjay Kumar for their valuable Suggestion, co-operation as well as well healthy criticism which make possible completion of this work.

Dr. Debasish Kundu
Dr. Ajit Singh

Contents

1 Chapter

Introduction to Electro Homoeopathic Pharmacy

The science of Electro Homeopathy was discovered by Italian noble Count Cesare Mattei, whose work 'Vade Mecum of Electro Homeopathy' was published Paola Bertero in Castle Monferrato, in which Mattei says '*that it would seem to be alchemy, if he explained of what vegetal electricity really consists*' quoting on a particular range of his medicines. The word pharmacy is derived from the greek word "pharmakon', which means combining from denoting relationship to drug or medicine. It is a process of preparing the drugs, which includes sophistication in raw material analysis, analysis of chemical components, methods of preservation, combination and standarization of drugs, also, art of compounding and dispensing them.

The synonym of the word Pharmacist is 'Apothecaries'. The term Pharmaceuticals refers to the physical chemistry of drugs and clinical pharmacy. Electro homoeopathic pharmacy deals in particular art of preparation, preservation, combining and compounding the medicines used in the medical science of Electrohomeopathy.

The roots of Electrohomoeopathy Pharmacy are in Alchemy. What is Alchemy? It seems appropriate to ponder on what Alchemy might be and how this pondering can lead us to spiritual progress. At this point, it is perhaps easier to describe what alchemy is not, rather than what it is. From a material point of view, Alchemy is neither chemistry nor hyperchemistry, but a biodynamic process more closely related to fermentation or putrefaction than to classical chemical reactions. Alchemy leads to a profound knowledge of the fundamental mechanisms of nature, yet is contrary to profane science which only considers the material aspects of these mechanisms. Alchemy considers the spiritual aspect as well as which is generally invisible to the sensory perception of the operator. This aspect of alchemical study brings the operator to spiritual progress, to a higher level of consciousness. The duality of this method of spiritual advancement has a great advantage over other methods. Spiritual advancement "makes one high" but, in order to accomplish the work, the Alchemist must remain grounded. He becomes aware of higher realities while he keeps in mind the significance of physical manifestations.

What is the Difference Between Chemistry and Alchemy?

In chemistry, if we have the right ingredients and if operations are correctly performed, success will be achieved-independently of the operator.

In Alchemy, even if we have the right ingredients and if operations are properly conducted, success is not necessarily achieved because it depends upon the personal state of the operator. In a very restrictive sense, Alchemy could be viewed as the paraphysiology of chemistry, for the success of the operation depends upon the inner spiritual state of the operator.

The second difference between the Chemistry and Alchemy is also important. Chemistry doesn't view the bodies it works with as alive. As a matter of fact, the processes are such that chemistry only deals with dead bodies which, of course, can't evolve. Conversely, Alchemy is a biodynamic system which uses the forces of life in its operation. A threefold work is accomplished on bodies: the effects are purification, regeneration and evolution. The most powerful principle are found in the forces of fecundation and reproduction and from these they will be extracted in order to be used. But if this operation seems possible in the vegetable realm, the extraction of the metallic semen or sperm, known only be a few adepts, is considered a Utopian venture by most. The Alchemist or the skilled artist can and must accomplish, through physical material, the manipulation of the divine, spiritual and invisible components which are, in beings and things, the genuine elements of life. According to Mattei (founder of Electrohomoeopathy) the cause of every illness lay hidden in two bodily fluids, the Blood and Lymph. The two fluids are responsible not only for transporting nutritive matter but also the seat of immaterial powers that circulated throughout our body. According to Mattei Electrohomoeopathy Pharamcy, A complete cure was atainable only through compound medicines whose components synergically complemented each other so as to increase their combined effect. That effect, however, was immaterial. Remedies worked, it was thought, by influencing the electric nature of the body's "Life force". In Electrohomoeopathy the life power is a synonymous to the word "Od" given by the Karl von Reichenbach (1788-1896). He described that the existence of a universal power that penetrated all things in the cosmos. The notion was a common one in occult circles in the nineteenth century and was often discussed in terms of aura, astral bodies, animal magnetism, or animal and vegetable electricity. Reichenbach thought that such energy could actually be seen by "sensitive" individuals in the form of light radiation from objects in a darkened room. He called such appearances "Od" after the all piercing power of the Germanics God Odin. Mattei referred the same energy as a "life force". The force was universal in its effect and formed the metaphysical basis for an interaction between animate and inanimate matter. Just as the human body maintains itself through an exchange of nutritive matter, Mattei and his disciples reasoned, there must also take place within every organ a circulation of nutritive energy. Such an energy, or "life force" had its origins in the large world. For terrestrial things, its main source via the sun.

Mattei believed he had perfected the empirically based homeopathic procedures first described by Hahnemann. From a shrub that he obtained in the Apennines, Mattei extracted what he called a vegetable electricity. This notion, i.e. the idea of vegetable electricity, and the assumption that many of his preparations worked as fast as the flow of an electric current, were primarily responsible for the name "ELECTRO-HOMOEOPATHY". In its full glory the system of Electrohomoeopathy is quite complex, nevertheless, in each case the aim of treatment is not the combating of symptoms or even individual illness, but the restoration of the function of organs through a power exchange in the body that involved the transmission of "Od" like energies. Medicines, most derived from the plants, are administered as globules or in dilutions as well also employed, largely for external use, medicinal liquids that assisted the circulation of the "life force" and correspond to the "fluid of the nerves". The first quantitative references to electrohomoeopathic medicines appeared in 1919, while a classifiaction of remedies was supplied by one of Mattei's successors, Theodor Krauss. The Electrohomoeopathy medicines are called Spagyric Medicine. Spagyric is a unique and harmonious blend of herbal medicine, homeopathy, aromatherapy and mineral therapy for holistic healing, a therapeutic treatment that heals body, soul, and the spirit at the same time. Unlike other natural therapies,it focuses on the real cause of the ailment, making it possible to understand why a person became ill and thus leading to a more complete healing. This idea is also the foundation of ancient therapeutic ways of healing, such as traditional Chinese, Tibetan and Ayurvedic medicines. Spagyric presents to modern practitioners a large variety of remedies for all facets of human ailments. In contrast with traditional plant remedies, spagyric is totally non toxic and without any side effects.

Paracelsus (1493-1541) discovered the Spagyric process for preparing a healing essence made up of all the components of a plant. He coined the word "spagyric" from two Greek words meaning "separate" and "reunite", alluding to the specific preparation process of a spagyric essence. During this process, the constituents of the plant will be separated, transformed, purified and recombined by methods inspired by Alchemy concepts. The resulting spagyric essence is natural and pure and possess a full spectrum of healing properties for the entire human being. The main difference between a spagyric essence and "classic" herbal tincture is the immaterial healing force developed in the production process of a spagyric remedy. This leads to a higher grade of efficiency, similar to the potential claimed in Homeopathy. One day quantum physics will emerge as a clue to understand that how the energy medicine works and how it is able to correct ailments for which allopathic medicines offer no answer.

Electrohomoeopathy Pharamcy Includes:

1. **Collection:** It is the gathering of the required drug materials. Exotic drug materials are imported from abroad if there substitutes are not available in the concerned country.
2. **Identification:** By mean of a Botanist, a drug must be examined microscopically as well as chemically too.
3. **Quality Inspection:** Proper physical and analytical procedures must be done to ascertain the quality of drugs, with the aid of suitable instruments and reagents and by chromatography too.
4. **Preserving:** if necessary, drugs and medicinal preparation should be properly preserved in accordance with their properties.
5. **Standardization:** Drugs so prepared are made to conform some standards as per the procedure given by the approved scientific committee.

6. **Combining:** Process of joining two or more things together in a scientific way.
7. **Compounding:** The method of uniting two or more different elements or constituents together so as to form an altogether new product. This new product will have new properties different from those of its constituents. This will produce a "Chemical Compound Mixture".
8. **Preparation:** In Electrohomoeopathy it includes the preparation of Spagyric Medicines, which further includes the preparation of Dilutions.
9. **Quality Control:** It reveals that whether the drugs and the medicines, so prepared from the ingredients are up to the standard so prescribed in the official Pharmacopeia. As well as it also includes the use of standard equipments and laboratory space and environment and preservation of drug and medicine. As well as it also includes the use of standard equipments, laboratory space, environment and preservation of drugs and medicines.
10. **Dispensing:** It means preparing and serving the medicinal preparation in accurate way according to the directions of qualified physicians.

What is Pharmacodynamics and Pharmacopoeia?

Pharmacodynamics is a study of the information about the interaction of the drug molecules and the body or may be said as the molecule which is carrying pharmacological message to the body.

Pharmacopoeia means the standard book containing a list of drugs and medicines, information about the sources, habitats, descriptions, collections and identifications of the drugs; and also provide directions for their preparation, combining, compounding and standardisation.

2 Chapter

Laboratory Equipments Used in Electrohomoeopathy Pharmacy

An Electrohomoeopathy Laboratory should be spacious enough providing Separate departments:

1. Manufacturing
2. Bonded Laboratory
3. Analytical Laboratory
4. Cloak rooms
5. Finished Products
6. Packing Departments
7. Administration.

In addition to these there should also remain sufficient space required for inter-departmental free movement. The laboratory should be provided with burning gas, electricity and enough quantity of water for washing and cleaning purposes.

List of General Equipments:

a. Coffee filter paper b. Cotton balls

c. Parafin

d. Quart Amber bottle

e. Quart Corning Glass pot

f. Faucet Adapter

g. Clamps

h. Stands

i. Coors porcelain crucible

j. Funnels assorted sizes

k. Glass stir rods

l. Graduated Glass Beaker

m. Kiln

n. Distillation Train

o. Mortar & Pestle

p. Portable electric stove

q. Soxhlet Extractor

r. Mason jars

s. Flasks

t. Test tubes

u. Misc. equipments as per requirement.

v. Microscopes

In a laboratory, evaluation data is generated, measured, calculated or assessed by automatic, mechanical or electronic or computerised equipment. The equipment should be of appropriate design and of adequate capacity to function according to protocols. Examples of such equipments include balances; calorimeters; spectrophotometers; pH meters; refractometer; analytical equipment computerised equipment for direct capture of data. The equipment should be suitably located for operation, inspection, cleaning and maintenance. It is to be assured that the equipments are performing their intended functions. The equipment should undergo validation process for proper functioning.

3 Chapter

Vehicles Used in Electrohomoeopathy

The meaning of term “vehicle’ is “means of conveyanace or transmission”. In electrohomoeopathy vehicles are the substances, in which medicines are prepared or mixed and provided for administrations by mean of internal or external application.

Vehicles are an inert substance having no therapeutic value which is used in the preparation of spagyric essence. In electrohomoeopathy the vehicles are used in preparation of tincture Aqueous fortis (Spagyric preparation of medicinal plants) or the preparation of different dilutions of requisite medicines and in external application. Vehicles are of dry and fluid constancies.

An ideal Vehicle

1. It must not have any medicinal property of its own.
2. It should be chemically neutral; neither acidic nor alkaline in medicinal effects. They must not undergo any change or decomposition.
3. The above two specific properties are more applicable to those which are used in potentising medicines.
4. It must be harmless regarding its action on human organisms. The pharmacological message of the original drug is not disturbed in any way.
5. It should be capable of carrying the dynamic powers of drugs into interior human organisms to fight the disease force.
6. It should be edible and palatable.

Liquid Vehicles

They are used for substances easily soluble in water or alcohol and for juicy substances. Solid triturations are converted into liquid potency with alcohol and water, as alcohol has a preservative virtue for keeping it for a longer period.

In Electrohomoeopathy, liquid vehicles used are:

I. Aqua Distillata (Distilled water).

Distilled Water

Mainly used in external applications. (Distilled Water or Aqua Distillata)

Chemical Formula-H2O Molecular weight/ Boiling point (B.P.)-IOO°C at 760 mm. of pressure; Freezing point (F.P.)-O° Critical Temp.-374 °C

At 4 degree celcius 1 ml water weight is 1 gmpH-Neutral; Density 1000 kg/m3. It is a very good solvent, having a physiological inertness, and is one of the most important vehicle used in Electrohomoeopathic pharmacy. There are three degrees of purity, e.g. 'Ordinary water ', 'purified water' and 'water for injection'. In Electrohomoeopathy properly purified water may also be used; which should be freshly prepared for use, and be sterile. It must be free from all bacteria and micro-organism.

Chapter 4

Sources of Electro Homoeopathic Medicines

Electrohomoeopathic medicines are prepared from both exotic & indigenious herbal medicinal plants, which grows in their natural habitats. The flowers, leaves, fruits, buds, roots & barks, etc are collected at the time of their maturity to obtain their highest medicinal contents. The plants are examined for contamination, such as other plants, insects or environmental pollution. Selected plants or parts are used in the preparation of spagyric medicines.

Some of the sources of the Electrohomeopathic medicines are given below:

1. **Whole plants (including root):** Aconitum napellus,Atropa belladonna, Matricaria, Chamomila, Chelidonium majus, Solanum, Dulcamara, Euphrasia officinalis, Ledum palustre, Pulsatilla nigricans, Ruta graveolens.
2. **Root:** Armoracia sativa, Cimicifuga racemosa, Hydrastis canadensis, Caphaelis ipecaauanha.
3. **Stem:** Caulophyllum thalictroides, podophyllum peltatum, Sanguinaria canadensis.
4. **Bulb:** Allium cepa, Allium sativum.
5. **Leavas:** Rhus toxicodendron, Artemisia, Abrotanum.
6. **Spores:** Lycopodium clavatum.
7. **Bark:** Euonymus europea, Berberis vulgaris.

The plants are collected soon as they attain their highest contents of active ingredients.

The plants should be free from insecticides, insect contamination or industrial pollution.

The optimum quality & purity of the plants are ensured through morphological, microscopical & phytochemical examinations.

5 Chapter

Collection of Medicinal Plants

The sources of Electrohomeopathic medicines is vegetable kingdom. Plants grown under constant supervision of trained personnel or grown in their natural habitat are collected as soon as they attain their highest contents of active ingredients.

These are graded, inspected & processed upon arrival at the laboratory to retain their freshness as well as the active medicinal contents in their native & stabilized form.

1. **Whole plants (including roots):** These are collected in sunny weather when these are in half flowering & half bud stage.
2. **Leaves:** These are collected before the flowering of the plants. In case of biennial herbs the leaves are collected in the spring time of second year, before the flowers develop from the buds.
3. **Flowers:** These are collected in dry weather, when these are partly in bud & partly in the blossom.
4. **Stems:** These are collected when most of the leaves of the plants are fully developed.
5. **Barks:** These are collected in the early spring for resinous herbs, & for the non resinous herbs, in the autumn.
6. **Roots:** These are collected in the spring in case of biennial herbs, when these are in their full vigour. In case of annual herbs, these are collected early in the autumn, before the ripening of the seeds & from perennial herbs these are

collected in the second or third year before the woody fibres develop in them.

6 Chapter

Cohobation: An Extraordinary Pharmacy

Cohobation in "Alchemy" is the assembling of the purified elements got by mean of spagyrism. It is not concern to the act of passing again and again a solvent over a substance to openit and to dissolve it as per the definition given by Glaser's.

Thus the process of reassembling the three purified principles (Salt + Sulphur + Mercury) constituted COHOBATION.

In alchemy, the meaning of words often has no sense with the meaning usually given to them. The three principles sulphur, mercury and salt have nothing in common with what is generally understood by these words.

All things & all beings possess Sulphur, Mercury, and Salt: these are principles which concentrate spiritual energies. The sulphur concentrate the soul's energies, the mercury the spirit energies & the salt the body energies.

Before cohobating these three principles, have to separate which is always known as the great secret of the spagyrism & alchemy.

In vegetable realm, the spirit is contained in the Alcohol & is common to all plants and released by all plants during the fermentation process (death) of the body. The spirit/Mercury is the life force of the cosmos & its vital essence & represents the major points of interest in Alchemy. The soul of the vegetable world is the essential oil which are plants possess to various degree. The soul (sulphur) is the consciousness of three world (kingdom). The Body (salt) of the vegetable world is what remaining after the spirit has left. It is also called caput-mortem (dead Head). It is than burnt until it turns into ashes and finally to white salt.

Cohobation is certainly is the delicate operation. However, if the sulphur & the salt have been purified, the cohobation between then occurs equal weight to equal weight. As for the Mercury, it should only imbibe the others two. Only by carefully watching the process, we can justify that if there is too much or too little mercury.

Various alchemists failed in there experiments for the simple reason because they do not know the theory or do not understand what is happening during experiments. We never get the desired results if we deals the alchemy as applying a cookbook. When we don't understand, what we are doing, we kill the subtle principles & we move from alchemy back to chemistry.

What is the difference between an Allopathic remedy and Spagyric Elixir?

In most cases, the making of allopathic remedies follows the classical method & thus spagyric sulphur & mercury are expelled out (eliminated). The remainder is what, in spagyrics, is called salt. Therefore such remedies can act on the material aspects, the Body, but in no way it can act on the Person's psyche, that is the spiritual aspect. Spagyric elixirs, on the other hand, retain the three principles & though his own action, the spagyrist does his best to keep them. Thus, it is the "soul medicine" which contains both negative body elements & positive elements of life.

There are three levels of the Living body, i.e. Material or Molecular level, the Information level, & the spiritual level. Spagyric medicines alone is consisting the three principles, and the perfect medicine in the world to act on the three mentioned levels of the body.

As per Dr. V. Bott (author of Anthropolosophical Medicine) there is also connection between alchemical & homoeopathic concepts; both defy the concepts of Cartesian logic.

Let's recall two essential principle of homoeopathy.

1. After the dilution the product must be energized, that is to say the product must be energetically successes by hand.
2. Since a decimal dilution is a dilution by 10, we could logically think that two decimal dilutions: 1x1 = 1 are equal to the dilution 1C that is 1.

Well, this is wrong. A sequence of homoeopathic dilution provokes the inversion of the effects of the remedy but this inversion occurs often the same numbers of dilutions, whether they are decimal or centesimal.

1. For the two or three first dilutions, the product remains toxic.
2. From the third to the tenth or eleventh dilution, the product is curative.
3. From the eleventh or twelve dilutions to the fourteenth dilution, it is again toxic.

In homoeopathic remedies, the dynamisation is what brings the force to the product. The product is neither a pure product nor a product regenerated by its division first into sulphur, salt & mercury & the reconstituted through COHOBATION.

The alchemical decomposition & recomposition eliminate the toxic impurities of the product & this operation brings in one operation a force that a long sequence of dynamisation couldn't bring.

This is why the alchemical elements should be diluted only once but in a big way: from one to twenty drops in a glass of a suitable liquid. It is also very important in these elixirs by a sequence of homoeopathic successions.

In alchemy after the Cohobation the product undergoes a long Digestion at a constant temperature or a circulation. According to Von Bernus definition, the aim & the effect of digestion is to obtain the loosening of the textures of substances to allow their opening & dissolution. This phenomenon must be considered as identical to the one that happens in the stomach of an animal.

As per Dennis William Hauck, 'Cohobation' is a distillation process after 'digestion'.

"The plant's soul (or Sulfur) is obtained by steam-distilling the essential oil from the crushed plant. The remaining parts of the plant are digested and fermented, and the resulting solution is rectified to get the alcohol or spirit of Mercury, which is its life force. The residue of stems and leaves left behind is the plant's dead body. This material is dried and incinerated to ash. The ash is ground fine, dissolved in water, and filtered. The liquid is then evaporated, which produces a fine, white crystalline Salt. This is the plant's true body. The separated Three Essentials are now recombined. First, the crystallized Salt is roasted for a week. Then the Salt is ground again and spread in a warm dish outdoors to absorb atmospheric moisture. Alternatively, a few drops of fresh dew can be added. This whole process is repeated two more times. Next, the Salt is saturated with its oily Sulfur and placed in an incubator. After a week, the Salt is reanimated by saturation with the alcohol spirit of its Mercury. After a period of digestion, the solution is distilled by cohobation, in which the condensate is poured again and again upon the matter left at the bottom of the vessel. Finally, the original plant is resurrected in an exalted form known as the elixir."

As per Theodore Krauss cohobation is a cold distillation process with fermentation that retained the living, radio-active powers of the plants by accumulating or suspending them in the obtained essence. He recommended to gather the shoots, seeds, branches, leaves, blossoms, fruit, bark, bulbs or roots of the plants one needed in the spring or autumn, when the juices of the plant organism were active, extract their juices by making incisions and soak them in distilled water (maceration) at 35 °C. After that, one had to keep macerating fresh plant material, not in water, but in that solution. The solution gained more and more medicinal substance in the process until full saturation was achieved. The tincture should then be poured into big glass containers, called recipients, where it remained until it was completely clear; as a result of the fermenting process the impure substances would settle on the ground of the recipient as sludge, while the pure, clear essence contained all the medicinal properties of the plant in a refined, "virtually spiritualised" form, but without the ballast of the plant body and only bound to a small amount of water. (*Pathways of Homoeopathic Medicine*: Bettina Blessing, Institute for the History of Medicine, Robert Bosch Foundation, Stuttgart, Germany).

According to Clare Goodrick-Clarke, to perform Cohobation, the purified salts are placed in a huge jar and the tincture is poured over them. There will be a distinct change in the color and aroma of the mixture. The jar is to be sealed tightly, and placed in a warm, dark place and left for two weeks, then the solution is to be decanted into a dark glass bottle, which is the spagyric tincture, "It is good medicine in its own right, but one final step will make it even better: In this next phase, which is called exaltation, sublimation, or simply circulation, the tincture is dynamized into a true essence." (*Alchemical Medicine for the 21st Century*: Spagyrics for Detox, Healing, and and Longevity By Clare Goodrick-Clarke, Chapter 6, p. 104)

As per Hermetic philosophy, Cohobation (elevation) is the rejoining of distillate to it's source for further distillation or co-habitation after marriage of the opposites or the three purified prima materials. Which is achieved through repeated distillations in which the distillate is repeatedly reunified with the residue, and the distillation is carried out a new. Through continual changes in the aggregate conditions of the distillate and through the reunification with the residue in the distillation container, the distillate attains a high level of purity and, at the same time, its effectiveness is dynamised. (Hermetic library article; "Spagyric Elixirs Pt. 3: Further Calcination and Cohobation").

In the webpages of revolvy.com (as on 16 September 2017), under the topic 'Cohobation' the following is written:

> "In pre-modern chemistry and alchemy, cohobation was the process of repeated distillation of the same matter, with the liquid drawn from it; that liquid being poured again and again upon the matter left at the bottom of the vessel.[1] Cohobation is a kind of circulation, only differing from it in this, that the liquid is drawn off in cohobation, as in common distillation, and thrown back again; whereas in circulation, it rises and falls in the same vessel, without ever being drawn out.[2] [3]
>
> Cohobation has no corresponding process in modern chemistry, as it is not a useful process. Indeed, it is equivalent to performing the same distillation a number of times and does not increase the purity of the distillate or alter the residue any more than would be done by maintaining it at elevated temperature for the same period of time. The Dean-Stark trap does involve returning some distillate to the reaction flask: a solution is distilled and the condensed liquid is collected in a tube wherein water settles to the bottom and is drained out, while an organic solvent returns to the boiling solution. However, the process is not manual, most of the solvent does not leave the reaction flask, and the apparatus achieves a useful purpose (removing water from the reaction mixture). Circulation, on the other hand, is approximately the same as

reflux, where a solution is maintained at its boiling point by condensing the distilling vapors and returning them directly to the reaction mixture."

References

1. "Cohobate"; "Cohobation". Oxford English Dictionary. Oxford University Press. 2nd ed. 1989.

2. This article incorporates text from a publication now in the public domain: Chambers, Ephraim, ed. (1728). "Cohobation". Cyclopædia, or an Universal Dictionary of Arts and Sciences (first ed.). James and John Knapton, et al.

3. This article incorporates text from a work in the public domain: Porter, Noah, ed. (1913). "Cohobation". Webster's Dictionary. Springfield, Massachusetts: C. & G. Merriam Co.

7 Chapter

Methods of Prepartion of Spagyric Medicines

The roots of the spagyric or spagyrism can be traced back to thousands of years, a founder can not clearly be defined. The word spagyric was used often synonymously to the term "Alchemic". Spagyric is to be received rather a special branch of Alchemy with which in a special manufacturing process the welfare plant is unlocked and/or transformed.

The spagyric method is of separation, purification & reunification (Cohobation), it is constituted with the etymology of the Greek word spagiry (Spao+ageiro) which means to separate and reunite.

Spagyric medicines were originally created by fermenting parts of the wild herbs. This process produced concentrated aromatic solutions that were extracted and separated from the bulk plant matter. After fermentation was completed the,

1. Plant material was distilled in a special device
2. And the remainder dried & burned up.
3. The ashes were extracted and purified via distillation, than recombined with the concentrated solution.
4. As a result the finished spagyric essence contained the mineral constituent parts of the plants.

A spagyric essence is clearly colorless to yellowish and smells very intensively aromatically.

The nature of spagyric essences is subtler than that of spagyric tinctures. They are less 'Corporeal' more 'Dematerialized' & their effects is more penetrating but very subtle. Everything is subtler than with the extracts or even tinctures. Spagyric essences are therefore considered pure medicines.

Spagyric essences have a much longer life span; a virtually unlimited life span .as for their preparation much experience is required in the art of distillation.

Production of Spagyric Essence

All preparation always contains the three philosophical principles.

1. Mercury
2. Sulphur
3. Salt

These principles are extracted (separation), purified (distillation, incineration, calcinations, evaporation) & then reassembled (reunion or Cohobation).

The practical works of the alchemy lab whether we mean the inner or outer lab-includes three basic process, i. e. separation, purification, and cohobation. These three processes are the basis of the evolutionary process of all alchemical works.

In nature, whenever a plant dies, its body is biodegraded and its essential principles (sulphur +mercury+ salt) returns to the earth to be used in the life cycle of other plants. The cycle remain in circulation unless an animal eats the plant, in which case the vibration of the plant are transmitted to a higher level by the alchemical power of the living animal realm. This is an internal or naturally happening to this planet.

But if externally or in the alchemical lab, an herb is separated into its essential principle, the oil, the alcohol & the caput-mortem. Each Principle is then purified by using heat (the fire) through distillation, extractions and calcinations. The final step is Cohobation which represents a rebirth on a higher level. Thus the plant is taken out of the bio-degradation cycle and is reborn through the raising of its vibration to a level where it can be used for a higher purpose that is medicine in animal realm.

The medicines which are produced through alchemical methods are more efficient than any other vegetable medicine because they contain the three essential principles in a purified & cohobated state.

Steps to be followed to get the Spagyric Essence

(Reunification of alchemy Sulphur, Mercury & Salt)

Extraction of Sulphur (Volatile oils):

1. Steam distillation performed to the crude drug to obtain the volatile oils. Take a 5000 ml round bottom flask into a sand bath & poured 3000 ml of distilled water into the flask. Take another wide mouth double jointed flask and place a small piece of filter paper inside the flask over the bottom joint. Now add enough grounded herb to the flask so it is half full. Next, hook up the reduction head and the distillation adapter. At last use a 2000 ml flask as a receiver at the end of the apparatus.

2. Turn the heat on low after some time, steam will colored up the double-jointed flask as it passed through it. The distillation adapter also will become fogged. At the end of the drip tip there will we see that water droplets are forming. The drops will fall into the receiver. After few milliliters have collected in the receiver, there will be colored oil is collecting on top of the water and when approximately 1500ml of the water has been distilled off, turned off the heat and let the apparatus cool. Then transferr the water and oil in the receiver into the oil separator.

3. Took the double-jointed flask off of the distillation flask. Poured 100 ml of the fresh distilled water into the distillation flask & hook up the entire apparatus. This entire process should be done at least three times to ensure that the majority of the volatile oils come out of the plant body.

Collection of Oils

4. While the second separation of the sulphur is under way, gather the oils obtained from the first. To do this, simply open the stopcock t the end of the drain tube. Slowly drain off the water, when only a little water is left in the separator, close the stopcock. After each subsequent extraction of the volatile oils from the plant body, take what is in the receiver and place it in the oil separator leaving the oil behind. Reuse this water for all other subsequent separations of oil from the plant body.

Extraction of Mercury

5. Take the essence from the depleted body of the herb and place it into the wide mouthed 5000 ml round bottom flask. The water that was left from the separation of the volatile oils is now poured over the herb. Seal up the round bottom flask with a fermentation lock and placed it in an incubator at 27 degree centigrade. In about two weeks, the plant body will have fermented and yielded up its spirit i.e. Mercury. Distilled off the spirit as done before and rectified it seven times. Save the phlegm from the spirit for later use.

Extraction of Salt

6. Take a glass pot & empty the remaining liquid and plant body left in 5000 ml flask. Take the pot out door and boil off all the moistures. When the moisture is gone, the herb body will begin to roast, than incinerate it. When the body will obtain an ash grey color, turn off the heat & let the pot cool. Grind and weigh the ash set up the soxhelt extraction & extract the water-soluble salts from the ash. Evaporate

the water from the salts in the oven overnight. Grind and weigh the salts, than place them into the kiln to calcine at 600 degree centigrade for one week. At the end of the week, turn the kiln off and let it cool. Grind & weigh the salts. Repeat the process of extracting, drying, grinding, weighing, claiming, grinding and weighing two more times to get the hygroscopic salt, the third principle (ingredient).

Cohobation

7. Once got hygroscopic salt, now it is time for cohobation, mix rectified spirit i.e. Mercury (already preserved) the salt then add the volatile oils i.e. Sulphur.

Digestion

8. Allow the mixture to digest in an incubator at 30 degree centigrade for a week. Be sure to slightly shake the container three to five times a day.

Decantation

9. Decant the essence (spagyric essence) from the undissolved salts. It will be seen that the essence is now colored yellow and smells strongly of the herb been used in the operation.
10. One drop in wine or distilled water will yield the full effects of the plant's medicinal nature. Save the remaining salt.
11. The essence is further used for medicinal preparation which is higher in its quality & non toxic in nature.

In existing age the Electro homoeopathy medicine producing in the name of Homoeopathy in Germany by a company ISO- Arzneimittel.

In Germany the Electro complex mode of treatment known as spagyric according to Kraus (one of the great follower of Mattei). It is a part of the official German Homoeopathic Pharmacopoeia. In this form this treatment is accepted by the Government of Germany. The Products produced by ISO-Arzneimittel sold to Germany, England, Italy, Spain, USA, Pakistan, India, and Sweden.

The Spagyric Medicine produced by the ISO-Arznemittel are constituted as the spagiric manufacturing process after Krauss, according to this:

"The Spagiri words leads itself from the Greek "spao"= separates & "ageirein"=combine off. Related to the medicament production, this means the separation of the valuable one from the "Impure one". This separation takes place in the JSO Complex Heilweisen particularly carefully in two steps.

1. The fermentation of the vegetable raw material and
2. An alcoholic extraction of the remaining firm components.

After two separate exponentiation steps the two excerpts in the third power are combined (agerein). The characteristics of the spagyric dressing after Krauss are:

a. The exclusive use of vegetable material.
b. The careful dressing.
c. The use of alcohol and water soluble contents materials.
d. The avoidance of toxicological side effect by the exponentiation of the components.

The process adopted by the ISO- Arzneimittel Germany is less spagyric or not a true spagyric. Because only some of the plant's salts dissolve in ethanol, specifically those of mineral characteristics. Organic salts are not generally soluble through maceration, which, could only be collected through calcination.

"Spagirik" to Krauss (ISO Arzneimittel GmbH, Ettlingen): Theodor Krauß (1864-1924) developed a drug system called "Spagirik" with the pharmacist Johannes Sonntag after the First World War, but apart from the fermentation this method does not use any of the traditional spagyric techniques. (*Spagyric Healing*-By Ulrich Arndt, Ernst-Moritz-Arndt-Universität Greifswald, Germany).

Similarly, some more Germany school following another method:

* A soxhlet extractor is filled with the chosen plant.
* The menstruum used is distilled water.
* Perform three cycles of extraction. As water is not bothered by the presence of alcohol.

After the three cycles, allow it cool down & carefully pour from the condenser side an equal quantity of 96% alcohol and water for a 200 ml-300 ml water soxhelt there is then in the flask 600 ml of a mix and half of it is alcohol. In fact if now provide a little heat, the alcohol alone is going to pass and got an extraction of the tincture which occurs rather quickly in three cycles.

When this is finished, the solid residue of the thimble is claimed at a high temperature; 1200°C minimum, even 1600°C is sometimes preferable. The residual ash is thrown into the menstruum while very hot & the whole is put to maceration for a week. Then a simple filtering yields the spagiric.

But here it is contrary to the alchemy, there are no clear salt- tincture separation and no separation sulphur-mercury at all. The salt is not charged with sulphur, but it simply has the role of absorbing impurities of the tincture.

The German school which uses this process does not intend to join the alchemical path through it. It remains within the framework of healing authorized by laws of the country. So the purpose of giving example just to prove that how the wrong methods are in bloom rather there is a difference between typical alchemical and papyri process.

A Few Rules to Follow in Laboratory

(Safety in laboratory)

1. Know the theory of the experiment we are considering. Do not attempt anything at random.

2. Study the properties of the products going to be produced or have to use in the production prior to the Experiment.
3. Operator's safety in the laboratory:
   - respect the safety regulation for gas, electricity etc,
   - never eat, drink or smoke in the laboratory,
   - always wear glasses.
4. Wear water proof rubber gloves which will protect us while handling acid or alkali liquids.
5. Wear asbestos gloves to handle molten liquids.
6. Wear asbestos gloves over the rubber gloves when handling acids or bases and hot liquids.
7. Wear leather or water- proof plastic shoes, no cloth or perforated shoes.
8. Have a working fire–extinguisher and a container filled with cold water close at hand. If there is an electrical heating system, make sure that the extinguisher is designed to extinguish electrical fires.
9. Mix unknown liquids in small quantity only. Always proceed as follows: pour a small amount of liquid in a test tube and a little bit of the other liquid into another test tube, close & keep the tubes away from each other. Mix the contents of the tubes slowly & must wear glasses when doing such kind of job.
10. Never pour a cold liquid in a hot liquid & vice versa.
11. Never pour water into an acid.
12. Permanent ventilation of the laboratory:
    - in case of the use of solvent
    - in case of gas heating
    - fume hood for dangerous gases.
    - no flames during work with volatile liquids.

13. The use of electrical heating is preferable during the handling of volatile liquids.
14. Never smell directly from a flask just wave a little.
15. Place wire gauze between the flask & the gas flame.
16. Never distill to dryness bodies giving peroxide, ether, acids etc. only water and alcohol can be distilled to dryness.
17. As much as possible, avoid any contact between rubber or cork stoppers and the extraction liquids.
18. Never force to join ground glass tubes.
19. Never exert mechanical force on glass welds.
20. Wet the flexible tubes (rubber or plastic) to be slipped on the glass.
21. Use cork or waxed- cork stoppers for distilled water or sulphur- free rubber stoppers.
22. Grease the ground joints silicon grease before joining. If a ground glass joint stick, try to pull the two parts apart, by hammering lightly on the ground joint with a plastic tool; if this too not work lightly heat the ground joint or use hot water.
23. To clean the glassware, rinse the flasks with ethyl alcohol, then with liquid detergent, followed with regular powder and then with clear water. Finish with a light rinse with distilled water or dematerialized water or dry the inside of the flask.
24. Bleach is excellent in all care, particularly to clean up calcinations residues. It must be less than three months old. Never bleach in contact with acid otherwise chlorine very toxic gas is given off.

8 Chapter

Quality Control Procedures

Modern laboratory procedures of quality control do not invalidate Cesare Mattei's original precepts nor replace classical procedures.

Indeed, had modern advances in scientific knowledge and equipment been available to Ceasor Mattei, he, in his wisdom would certainly have taken advantage of them. It must be emphasized, however, that ultimately the attainment of a high quality standard is only possible if one could rely on the integrity, involvement, training, and the commitment of all concerned. This is essentially a team activity with the objective to guarantee the purity, reliability and reproductability supplied to the practitioners.

It must be emphasized, however that ultimately that attainment of a high quality standard is only possible if one could rely on the integrity, the involvement, the training and experience and the commitment of all concerned, and the objective must always be to guarantee the purity, reliability and reproductability of the medicines supplied to the practitioners of the healing art.

High standards of personal cleanliness must be maintained by all personnel and hand washing facilities made available and used at regular intervals.

Protective clothing including gloves and hat should be worn in manufacturing facilities not only by the manufacturing personnel but also by the visitors. Cleanliness and proper hyginic conditions are the primary requirements. Utensils are required to be thoroughly washed after every use.

Incoming raw materials should be transfered to a quarantine store on each delivery.

Each delivery is allocated a reference or batch number to identify the material in every stage of manufacture, samples are taken from every batch to carry out tests for raw material specifications. Specimens may be photographed in certain cases subjected to microstructure analysis from which micro photographs are taken. All raw materials are released from the quarantine store only after they are labelled as fit for use according to specifications. Rejected raw materials are stored separately for disposal. The finished products are packed and labelled subject to quality control inspections.

At every step of manufacturing all equipments are inspected to ensure that these are clean and free from all contaminations, all raw materials and equipments are carefully labelled to identify the material being processed and products are labelled at every stage with batch number, manufacturing procedure is strictly followed in each step of production and batch records are maintained indicating times, temperatures, weights, etc., so the history of every batch from raw materials used to labelling of finished products may be checked at a later date if necessary. At every step quality control personnel are required to make spot checkings and collect samples for laboratory analysis to ensure absolute quality control and thus purity of the products. On completion of manufacuring, representative samples of the products are taken and labelled with the batch number and identity. Analytical tests are carried out in the laboratory to ensure that the product meets the finished product specifications and thereafter the product is labelled as ready to despatch. Samples of each batch of the product is always retained in the laboratory. Storage conditions are carefully followed to ensure that the product does not deteriorate during transport or further storage at the stockists place.

General precautions for quality control include segregation of processing areas to avoid possible cross contamination, the use of laminar air flow equipment or air conditioners, and all operations including the segregation of processing areas to avoid any possible cross contamination, the use of laminar air flow or air conditioning and all operations are carried out in such a way that the risk of contamination is minimized. Microbiological testing by swab or settle plate method to monitor environmental contamination of the entire manufacturing area is recomneded. Areas to be tested include laboratory benches water taps, valves and toilets.

Physical Properties

Spagyric Essences and Tinctures may be routinely tasted for their physical properties, including specific gravity, refractive index, colour, smell and taste.

General Tests: These may include plant residue (prior to burning), pH levels, water and alcohol content. Karl Fischer technique is the prescribed method for determining the water content.

Chemical Analysis: Conventions chemical methods are to be followed which could provide a means of identification and a guide of the purity to the spagyric tinctures, this include a thorough analysis for mineral salts and trace elements.

Thin Layer Chromatography: It utilizes the different migration rates for individual constituents of spagyric tinctures on a thin film of inert material. It shows characteristic bands on a layer of silica gel of 25-250 cm thickness, each band representing a specific chemical constituent of the spagyric tincture itself, but different batches of the same spagyric tincture. Various solvents are used such as butanol/acetic acid or methanol/chloroform over development distances of about 10 cm. It is used widely throughout the world in preparation of herbal tinctures to ascertain the purity, reproducibility and therapeutic effectiveness of the end products.

VEGA point testing or other types of analysis make it possible to determine and compare the amount of inherent energy in remedies produced by Spagyric method. Here the huge qualitative advantages of spagyric remedies become obvious. Importantly, practitioners are able to experience the excellent efficacy of these Electro Homeopathic spagyric medications through the fast, lasting results produced in patients. If the excretion process is not stimulated, and the internal terrain not improved, then the ill body may be forced to store toxins in the connective tissues, or aid excretion by other means such as fever, diarrhoea, and excessive sweating. This can be avoided by using Electro Homeopathic remedies.

Electro Homoeopathic medication possesses the distinct advantage of being both a high-energy spagyric. These remedies stimulate with their spagyric phyto-components, which provide an extra energy boost and regulate via the Electro Homoeopathic properties of individual plant constituents. This powerful combination creates "super-charged" remedies that invigorate the body's vital energy, act as immune system catalysts and promote more efficient cellular activity to help infected or weakened organ tissues resume normal function.

Kirlian Photography

In 1939, Semyon Kirlian discovered by accident that if an object on a photographic plate is subjected to a high-voltage electric field, an image is created on the plate. The image looks like a colored halo or coronal discharge. This image is said to be a physical manifestation of the spiritual aura or "life force"which allegedly surrounds each living thing.

Allegedly, this special method of "photographing" objects is a gateway to the world of auras. Actually, what is recorded is due to quite natural phenomena such as pressure, electrical grounding, humidity and temperature. Changes in moisture (which may reflect changes in emotions), barometric pressure, and voltage, among other things, will produce different 'auras'.

Living things are moist. When the electricity enters the living object, it produces an area of gas ionization around the photographed object, assuming moisture is present on the object. This moisture is transferred from the subject to the emulsion surface of the photographic film and causes an alternation of the electric charge pattern on the film. If a photograph is taken in a vacuum, where no ionized gas is present, no Kirlian image appears. If the Kirlian image were due to some paranormal fundamental living energy field, it should not disappear in a simple vacuum (Hines 2003).

There have even been claims of Kirlian photography being able to capture "phantom limbs," e.g., when a leaf is placed on the plate and then torn in half and "photographed," the whole leaf shows up in the picture. This is not due to paranormal forces, however, but to fraud or to residues left from the initial impression of the whole leaf.

Parapsychologist Thelma Moss popularized Kirlian photography as a diagnostic medical tool with her books "*The Body Electric*" (1979) and "*The Probability of the Impossible*" (1983). She was convinced that the Kirlian process was an open door to the "bioenergy" of the astral body. Moss came to University of California, Los Angeles (UCLA) in mid-life and earned a doctorate in psychology. She experimented with and praised the effects of Lysergic Acid Diathylamide (LSD) and was in and out of therapy for a variety of psychological problems, but managed to overcome her personal travails and become a professor at UCLA's Neuropsychiatric Institute. Her studies focused on paranormal topics, such as auras, levitation and ghosts. One of her favorite subjects at UCLA was Uri Geller, whom she "photographed" several times. She even made several trips to the Soviet Union to consult with her paranormal colleagues. Moss died in 1997 at the age of 78.

Moss paved the way for other parapsychologists to speculate that Kirlian "photography" was parapsychology's Rosetta stone. They would now be able to understand such things as acupuncture, chi, orgone energy, telepathy, etc., as well as diagnose and cure whatever ails us. For example, Bio-Electrography claims to be a method of investigation for biological objects, based on the interpretation of the corona-discharge image obtained during exposure to a high-frequency, high-voltage electromagnetic field which is recorded either on photo paper or by modern video recording equipment. Its main use is as a fast, inexpensive and relatively non-invasive means for the diagnostic evaluation of physiological and psychological states.

Kirlian photography (aka corona discharge photography or spark electrography) has been shown to demonstrate an electrochemical image of pre- and post-adjustment with definite change in image.

Research has been conducted in the former USSR, and in Germany, China, and the U.S., among other countries, which supports the use of Kirlian photography to measure or assess vital force in living systems, and to evaluate treatment methodology. Kirlian photography is a technique of photographing the electrical discharge from an object when impressed with a high voltage field. It was discovered by Semyon Kirlian in Russia in 1939. The Russians have performed scores of experiments on live plants, animals, and humans with the Kirlian effect. Kirov State University of Kazakhstan has studied the Kirlian effect with electron microscopy. Supposedly the Kirov scientists saw the living "double" of a living organism in motion. Kirlian photography is best remembered for revealing a leaf which, a portion of it having been cut away, revealed the entire leaf in terms of its aura. This is described as the phantom leaf effect. The Russians observed that the high-frequency discharge seems to imply the existence of an elementary plasma-like constellation made of ionized excited electrons, protons, and perhaps other particles and giving off its own electromagnetic fields and the basis of biological fields. In 1968, Drs. Inyushin, Grishchenko, Vorobev, Shouiski, Fedorova and Gibadulin announced that "all living things—plants, animals and humans not only have a physical body made of atoms and molecules but also a counterpart body of energy which they termed the Biological Plasma body."

Life force can be conceptualized through the energetic body model. Research with Kirlian photography has been performed by very reputable scientists. Its application to clinical sciences is still very much in its infancy. Kirlian photography is considered safe but should not be used on people with pacemakers, heart disease, or during pregnancy.

The above discussion is to show that other healing arts and scientists have researched this technology. It is appropriate at this time that the Science of Electrohomoeopathy to look into this technology for future utilization especially to photograph the energy fields being transmitted by our medicines. Further serious study of this subject with research design methodology is encouraged.

9 Chapter

Pharmacodynamics of Electrohomoeopathy Essences

Minerals, trace elements and vitamins are the enablers of metabolism. Carbohydrates, proteins and fats needs them for their synthesis and degradation. The immune system needs them for proper functioning.

As per Biochemistry the human body contains some vital mineral salts, viz. calcium, phosphorus, magnesium, iron, sodium, potassium, fluorine, sulphur, chlorine and silicon a deficiency of which disturbs the functions or metabolism.

Trace elements are the activators and co-factors of enzymes and other regulatory molecules, they include selenium, copper, cobalt, iodine, iron, zinc, manganese, vanadium, chromium, boron, chlorine, silicon, fluoride, molybdenum, arsenic, germanium, lithium, nickel etc.

Trace elements and vitamins work in concert, they are inter-dependent. Effects of trace element deficiencies on living organisms are now accepted by scientists world wide, now a days, faulty agriculture with chemical fertilizers and pesticides, food processing losses and environmental pollution are the basic contributory factors leading to mineral salt deficiencies in living organisms.

Electro Homoeopathic Treatment in situations of Deficiencies. The active ingredients in Electro Homoeopathic Medicines are the mineral salts which function by stimulating neuro immuno endocrine system. The ways through this stimulation is brought about are:

i. By direct activation of certain pathways.

ii. By correcting malfunction in absorption, transportation and excretion.

iii. By redistributing mineral salts, trace elements, etc. which due to stress, disease or medication have become locked up in the wrong place, for instance, infection and cortisone treatment induce transport of zinc and iron to the liver, and the release of copper to the bloodstream, conditions or some signal or else may be lacking to restore normalcy. In oedema, sodium in excess quantity enter the cells. Electro Homoeopathic Medicines restores cell membrane integrity and restores proper absorption, transportation and excretion which are essential in accordance with 'transformation of matter' as per physiology.

iv. By compensating for a deficiency induced inactive pathway, it means redistributing any scare element to the tissues at potential risk or activating some alternative pathway, for instance, vitamin E and selenium have a number of overlapping roles, if vitamin E synthesis is stimulated, selenium deficiency would be less critical.

Many of our chronic diseases are actually caused due to excessive inflammation. Inflammation is initiated by the neutrophils, it's granules release cytotoxic metabolites aimed at destroying microbials and viral invaders, and by basophils to destroy allergens. Cytotoxic metabolites include peroxides and free radicals, these oxidising elements can also destroy the fatty acids that comprise cell membranes, causing necrosis of tissues in the inflammated area, their over activity is suppressed by anti oxidants produced by the cells. Anti-oxidants include the enzymes,vitamins A, E and C, zinc, copper and selenium, hence, these elements are required for the immune system or body's defence mechanism, the inflammatory attack and the healing of tissues. The special aspect of the spagyric technique followed in preparation of

Electro Homoeo Medicines is that importance is given to the mineral salts which are present in the plants grown in their natural habitats, as plants grown in different environments usually show a wide variation of mineral salt composition.

For instance, a plant grown in limestone soil would be expected to have a higher calcium content in comparison to the same plant grown in sandy soil. Analysis carried out by German and British Scientists has shown the presence of mineral salts like iron, calcium, sodium, sulphar, etc. and trace elements like zinc, potassium, copper, cobalt, selenium, magnesium and manganese in the medicinal plants.

In Biochemistry, mineral salt preparations are prescribed for therapeutic uses and as Physiologists have established salt-hunger or 'Chelation' causes ailments in human beings, The majority of mineral salts are soluble in water not in alcohol, so, even from the modern scientific view it will not be wrong to say Electro Homoeopathy is totally Scientific in which mineral salts produced in and from natural sources (in Biochemistry Chemically produced mineral salts are used throughout) in minute form is prescribed to relieve mineral salt deficiency or 'Chelation' in human body, thus to effect a far more natural and specific CURE.

Safety of Spagyric Medicines

Spagyric medicine are produced in such a way that no alkaloids or toxic molecules can be found in the final products. Though pure and undiluted their efficacy may be compared with the "highly diluted" homoeopathic remedies. They have no known side effects. The advantage of these spagyric essence that it consists therefore the fact that they contain organic and inorganic materials and very well compatible by small alcohol content and the dosage recommended on adherence to normal conditions. The active substances of the essence can be proven with modern analytic technology, both in quality and quantity.

Plant Life Concentrates contain a unique ability to:

- Alkalise the PH, neutralising acidity
- Remove many toxins and toxic molecules out of the body
- Cleanse and purify the liver within 28 days
- Oxygenate the cells, allowing more oxygen into the cells and brain
- Destroy harmful free radicals
- Rid body of harmful bacteria
- Purify and regulate the blood, effecting blood circulation and blood sugar levels
- Build the immune system
- Relieve pain caused by acidosis and inflammatory processes

We are far away from the system of similar and the pathogenesy of Hahneman. It is true that this system is attractive on the intellectual ground, but it is very easy to be lost in it, even for a confirmed homeopath.

The big dilemma, center of homoeopath discussions, is to know if we have to privilege or not a high dilution rather than a low dilution. it is wiped out, as far as spagyric is always turned to the composed and asserts that it is not necessary to dilute a substance to the infinite to increase its field and depth of action. The spagyric experience demonstrates that easily.

To finish, this bring us to raise an issue that takes us particularly to heart, the one of mineral elements, which are present as traces in spagyric essence. The presence of these micro nutrients or trace elements (area of the composed) flow directly and specifically from the spagyric way of preparation. Micro-nutrients (Cu,Zn,Si,Mg,etc.) have a considerable action as modifier or corrector of the field, as well on a structural point of view as plastic material, as on a functional point of view as bio-catalyst of enzymatic reaction necessary to any life.

To better understand, let we take only one example, the one of horsetail. The incorporation in the essence of soluble and insoluble salt contribute to considerably enrich its content in mineral salts (especially silica) and therefore it mineralizing power.

As a matter of fact, the vegetal spagyric elixir is characterized more than any other galien or homoeopathic pharmaceutical preparation by the extend of its range of action, which is located at three different levels;

1. Symptomatic Level (Sulphur)

Are of action of the herbal medicine and aromatherapy (Allopathy, short time effect and with limited duration, in relation with the presence of active principles (alkaloids, flavonoid, terpenes, etc.)

Here, it has to be noted the importance that spagyrists give to the problem of "vaporization of salts", formula that constitute in the modern chemistry, a total nonsence, by virtue of the steady character that is peculiar to the saline compound. The processes of salt vaporization constitute in the microcosm spagrico-alchemic, a major arcanum, preciously guarded. Any alchemist by dry way knows the importance of the nitrous and volatile salt of dew, that Altus, in the light of the precious comments of E.Canseliet, reveals charitably by process of fabrication. The analysis of this compund reveals the presence of sulphur inhibited with aerial niter. This sulphur increases the flux qualities of the salt in the melting pot, and adds in the medico-spagyric area removing toxicity properties to the vascular dilation and cardio-tonic properties.

2. Energetic Level (Mercury)

- Area of action of homoeopathy.

- Variable term of action

- In relation with the vibratory quality of the product and the receptivity of the patient.

3. Structural and Biocatalyst Level (Salt)

- Area of action of micro-nutritionist medicine (micro-nutrients)
- Duarable and in depth correction of the field
- Long term effects (several month)
- Reconstitution of the mineral reserves of the organism (Mg, si, Mn, Cu, Zn, Co....)

This repartition of sulphur, salt and mercury principles on the basis of Paracelsus Pharmacopoeia, is also the foundation of the holistic approach of the patient. Because if the spagyrics interested by the illness as a nosologic entity, it does not neglect to be interested like we have seen in the field that was favorable for the emergence of the illness.

Absorption of Spagyric Essences

The absorption of a drug involves its passage across cell membrane. The following factors played major role in absorption of the Electrohomoeopathy essences.

Physical State: Mostly essences are liquids so easily absorbed in compare to solids.

Particle Size: Essences are the energetic partcles as well as the trace elements and microelements so absorbed easily.

Solubility: Essences are in the form of solution, so easily absorbed in compare to solids.

Concentration: Spagyric essences are concentrated form therefore easily absorbed than dilute solution.

More about Spagyric Essences of Electrohomoeopathy

Q. *Are spagyric essences interfere with the prescriptions of other Doctrine?*

Ans. Spagyric medicine works hand in hand with any other remedies and will not interfere with the doctor's prescriptions or other allopathic or natural treatments but always keep the difference of 20 minutes in taking of different medicines.

Q. What sort of reactions can be expected?

Ans: It is possible sometime but not always to observe an exacerbation of symptoms in the few days after the beginning of the treatment, a skin reaction or an increase of pain. That is what we call in homoeopathy a therapeutic aggravation, a sign that the medication is well chosen, in this case, lower the dosage to the minimum and then increase it slowly. Dosage is individual and what seems appropriate for one person may not suit another. Listen to our body chemistry.

Q. When should the medicine be taken?

Ans: It should be taken before meals on an empty stomach, but it gives also good result if taken after meals. It is advised to keep the drops a few moments in the mouth before swallowing them.

Q. To drink coffee/tea/and to avoid mint is necessary?

Ans: There are no known interaction between these beverages and spagyric drops, but moderate consumption is recommended. A patient opting for a natural treatment is certainly concerned with his life style. Mint may be consumed, but not simultaneously with the spagyric drops.

Q. How the medicine can be stored?

Ans: Spagyric drops are delivered in pharmaceutical quality vials, which protects them from light. There is no need to store them in a refrigerated place, room temperature is ok (except in very hot weather). Natural preparations may change slightly after several months, a small deposits may appear, but it doesn't alter the quality of the preparation. In this case shake the bottle before use.

Q. What is the difference between spagyric medicine and homoeopathy or herbal medicines?

Ans: Herbal medicine are used to treat many physical ailments. Some plants may contain certain toxic active components and should be used only under the proper supervision of professionals.

Extracting the active principles of a material by a mixture of water and alcohol is the first step to make homoepathic remedies. The mineral elements of the plants are usually absent, a part of the healing potential of the original product is lost. This mother tincture, which can be very toxic depending on the plant or the substance, is then diluted according to a fixed protocol. Successive dilutions and succussions of this mother tincture create the homoeopathic remedies. The crux of homoeopathy is that the dilution of a toxic substance allows reversing its effects into a healing remedy.

On the other hand, spagyric essences are made from plants by a unique process, which neutralises their toxic components, but preserve their healing potential this rather complex process allows the extractions of all healing components of the plant (Essential oils, aromatic components, mineral and trace elements) and the same time transforms chemically the toxic components in non toxic ones, no alkaloids for instance are found in spagyric essences, the spagyric essence is more completed and complex extract than a mother tincture. It harbours the plant's energetic power and vital force. It is a concentrated extract, sometimes slightly coloured with typical flavours and smells. So the difference between spagyric and homoeopathy is even apparent to our senses, a homoeopathic remedy being hardly differentiated by smell or taste from a water-alchol solution. There is no reason to dilute this essence, as it is non toxic and already full of its healing potential. Spagyric is a complete medical system in itself. it is not only an energetic medicine like homeopathy but also an ever-evolving therapeutics, contrary to homoeopathy, considered by some to be medicine with frozen concepts.

10 Chapter

Dosages and Mode of Administration

Count Mattei advocated for one drop of essence or 2/3 medicated globules to be added in 2/3rd of a tumblerful (approx 250 ml) of distilled water to obtain the first dilution, successive dilutions are obtained by adding one teaspoonful of first dilution to 2/3rd of a tumblerful of distilled water, and so on.

To make dilutions in Centismal scale one part of essence is to be added to ninety-nine parts of distilled water, successive dilutions are made by adding one part of first dilution to ninety-nine parts of distilled water and so on.

Globules are medicated by pouring one drop of essence to a grain of no. 10 globules.

An intermediate dilution comes between the first and second dilution and is prepared by dissolving one globule in about 1 ml of water, and taken a tumblerful daily.

When two remedies are taken alternately the required dilution of each is prepared, half a glassful of one is taken in the morning and half a glassful of the other is taken in the afternoon, a teaspoonful of every 15/20 minutes.

Globules are taken dry on the tongue and allowed to dissolve naturally, the dosage is 1 globule half hourly, or else 8-10 globules are taken at a time depending upon the case.

External Application: Globules in dissolved form are used in baths, gargles, compresses, lotions, ointments, etc.

1. **Ointments:** These are prepared mixing the dissolved globules with olive oil or vaseline or glycerine.
2. **Baths:** For a full length bath, dissolve from 50 to 150 drops in a glass of warm water, and mix with the bath water-For sit-bath, dissolve from 25 to 50 drops-For foot-baths 15 to 25 drops.
3. **Compresses:** Dissolve 20 drops in about half-a-pint of water.
4. **For Gargles:** Dissolve 30 drops in a 6 ounce of water.
5. **Lotions:** Dissolve 20 drops in a little water, and add a tablespoonful of rectified spirits of wine. These lotions are applied by means of small sponge or soft brush to the head or scalp, or on the beard, applying it directly to the skin, or by rubbing the surface with a funnel.
6. **For Injections or Clysters:** 20 globules of the remedy prescribed, in a tumberful of distilled water.

11 Chapter

List of Medicinal Plants Used in Electrohomoeopathic Remedies

1. Artemisia abrotanum - Ang.-3
2. Arnica montana - Ang.-1, 3, Pett-4, Canc-6, W.E., App
3. Avena sativa - Ang.-1,2,3, W.E.
4. Aesculus hippocastanum - Ang.-2, Feb-1, 2, - Scrof 10
5. Achillea millefolium - Ang.-2, W.E.
6. Adiantium capillus veneries - Pett.-1,2,3,4
7. Alium cepa - Pett-1,2,3,4, Y.E.
8. Aloes capensis - Slass
9. Aconitum napellus - Feb.-1Pett-4, RE.
10. Ailanthus glandulosa - Canc-13
11. Althaea officinalis - Ven-1, G.E.
12. Atropa belladona - Scrof.-12, Canc-13
13. Allium sativaum - Verm-1, 2
14. Artemisia cina - Verm-1, 2
15. Agaricus muscarius - W.E.
16. Anthemis nobilis - W.E.
17. Berberis vulgaris - Feb .-1, 2 scrof .5, C1
18. Betula alba - Ven.-1
19. Capasella bursa pastoris - Ang. -1,B.E.
20. Cetraria islandica - Scrof. 10, Feb.-1,2, B.E.

21. Cinchona calisaya - Scrof. -10, Feb,-1,2, B.E.
22. Cinchona succirubra - Scrof .10, Feb. – 1, 2
23. Cimicifuga racemosa - Whit. Elect.
24. Conium maculatum - Canc.1,2,3,4,5.6,10, 13,15, 17 G.E.
25. Caulopphyllum thlictroides - Canc. -1
26. Carduus benedictus - Canc. -1
27. Chelidonum majus - Canc. -10, Y.E.
28. Cochlearia officinalis - Scrof.1,2,3,5,6,10,11,12,
29. Chenopodium anthelminiticum - Verm.-1
30. Cannabis sativa - Ven.-1
31. Clematis erecta - Ven.-1
32. Dictamnus albus - Verm.-1,2
33. Drosera rotundifoiia - Pett.-3
34. Daphne mezerum - Canc.-3
35. Eucalyptus globulus - Pett.-1,2,3,4, Ven.-1
36. Erythraea centsurium - Feb.-1,2, Scrof.- 10, Linf-1
37. Echinacea angustifiolia - Linf.-1
38. Euphorbium officinale - Verm.-1
39. Equisetum arvense - B.E.,G.E.
40. Ervum lens - Canc.-2(Pett.-2)
41. Euphrasia officinalis - Scrof.-12
42. Euonymus europaeus - A.P.P.
43. Fucus vesiculosus - Linf.-1
44. Gentiana lutea - Slass
45. Glechoma hederacea - Pett.-2
46. Galeopsis ochroleuca - Pett.-2
47. Genista scoparia - W.E.
48. Guajacum officinale - W.E.

49. Hyoscyamus niger - Pett.-3
50. Humulus lupulus - Linf.-1
51. Hamamelis virginica - Ang.-2, G.E.
52. Hydrastis canadensis - Ang.1,2,3 Pett-3, Scrof 1,2,3,5,6,10,12
53. Imperatoria ostruthium - Verm.-1
54. Lycopodium clavatum - Scrot .-2
55. Lobelia inflata - Scrof.-11
56. Ledum palustre - Canc.- 6
57. Marsdenia condurango - Canc.-15
58. Melissa officinalis - Scrof. -11
59. Myrthus communis - Ven.-1
60. Malva sylvestris - Ang.1,3
61. Menyanthes trifoliata - Linf.-1 ,W.E.
62. Matricaria chamonilla - Scrof. 1,2,3,5,6,11,12
63. Nasturtium officinale - Scrof.1,2,3,5,6,10,11,12
64. Oxalis acetosella - Linf.-1
65. Pulsatilla vulgaris - Ang.-3
66. Phelladrium aquaticum - Pett. 1,2,3,4
67. Petroselinum sativum - Canc.-2, W.E.
68. Phytalacca decandra - Canc.-5,G.E.
69. Podophyllum peltatum - Canc.-10Y.E.
70. Populus alba - G.E.
71. Papulus tremuloides - Canc.-17, Ven.-1, G.E.
72. Pinus nigra - B.E.A.P.P.
73. Pinus maritima - B.E.
74. Polygala amara - Pett-1,2,3,4
75. Pimpinella saxifrag - Canc.1,2,3,4,5,6, 10,13,15,17,
76. Pulmonaria officinalis - Linf.-1

77. Rheum officinale - Scrof-3
78. Rhus aromatica - Canc-17
79. Ruta graveolens - Verm- 1,2, W.E.Y.E.
80. Rosa canina - Ven-1, R.E.
81. Rhododendron ferrugineum - R.E.
82. Rosmarinus officanalis - R.E.
83. Rhus toxicodendron - Canc 1,2,3,4,5,6, 10,13,15,17,
84. Scrophularia nodosa - Scrof.,1,2,3,5,6,10, 11,12,A.P.P.
85. Solidago vigaurea - Scrof.- 6
86. Sambucus nigra - Feb.-1,2, Scrof.-10V.E.G.E.
87. Salix alba - Feb. -1,2, Scr0f .-10
88. Simaruba amara - Linf.-1
89. Smilax medica - Scrof.-1,2,3,5,6,10,11,12, Ven.-A.P.P
90. Sanguinaria canadensis - Ang.-1,2,3 W.E.
91. Scolopenderium vulgare - Feb.-2
92. Spigelia anthelmia - Verm.-2
93. Symphytum officinale - Canc.-4
94. Sanguisorba officinalis - W.E.
95. Salvia officinalis - B.E.
96. Salvia sclarea - B.E.
97. Solanum dulcamara - Ven-1
98. Strychnos nux vomica - Scrof.-1, Canc.-15, Slass
99. Steffensia elongata - Ven-1
100. Tussilago farfara - Scrof.-1,2,3,5, 6,10,11
101. Taxus baccata - W.E.
102. Teucrium scordium - Pett.2.

103. Thymus serpyllum	-	Verm.-1
104. Tanacetum vulgare	-	Verm.-2
105. Tilia europaea	-	Ven.-1
106. Thuja occidentalis	-	Ven.-1
107. Taraxacum officinale	-	W.E.,A.P.P.
108. Uragoga ipecauanha	-	Pett.-1,2,3,4,
109. Veronica officinalis	-	Scrof.-1,2,3,5,6,10,11, Ven.-1
110. Viburnum opulus	-	Ven.-1
111. Vinca minor	-	Ven.-1, A.P.P.
112. Viscum album	-	W.E.
113. Vitis vinifera	-	R.E., A.P.P.
114. Vincetoxicum officinale	-	Canc-1,2,3,4,5,6,10, 13,15,17

Note to the Readers:

Plant biology or phytology, genetics, ecology, distribution, classification, as well as pharmacological (i.e., chemical constituents) and therapeutic properties of all the above medicinal plants are dealt in greater details according to latest available informations in the book nos 9 and 12 listed in Bibliography at the end of this book, and available with the publisher of this book.

Appendix 1

Terminology

1. Ablation

The separation of a component by removing the upper part, sometimes by skimming it off the surface or by wicking it up using a feather or cloth.

2. Albification

The making of the matter in the alchemical work become white.

3. Ablution

The purification of a substance by successive washings with a liquid.

4. Alkaloids

They mean"Alkali-like". Alkaloids are organic bases, containing Nitrogen, having specific physiological actions. Vegetable alakoids occur in any part of plants,but are generally abundant in barks, seeds and roots.

5. Amalgamation

Formation of an amalgam, or alloy, of a metal with mercury. This term is sometimes extended to mean any union of metals.

6. Anhydrous

This term is applied to a substance, when it is completely free from water.

7. Ascension

When the active or subtle part rises up in the flask, usually by heating.

8. Assation

The reduction of a substance to a dry ash by roasting.

9. Bioavailablity

It is defined as the yield of the active drug from a pharmaceutical preparation at the required sites in the body.

10. Boiling Point

When a pure liquid boils under constant pressure and the temperature remains constant, then that constant temepertaure under one atomsphere sites in the body.

11. Calcination

The breaking down of a substance by fierce heating and burning usually in an open crucible.

12. Cementation

Acting upon a substance by mixing it in layers with a powdered (often corrosive) material, such as lime. This mixture is then be made to react and weld together by heating to a high temperature in a cementing furnace.

13. Ceration

The making of a substance to soften and appear like wax. This is often accomplished by continually adding a liquid and heating.

14. Cineration

The reduction of a substance to ashes by heating.

15. Circulation

The purification of a substance by a circular distillation in a pelican or closed distillation apparatus. Through heating the liquid component separates, is condensed and descends again to the substance in the flask.

16. Coadunation

Another term for coagulation.

17. Coagulation

The conversion of a thin liquid into a solid mixture through some inner change, as with the curdling of milk. This can be accomplished by a variety of means - by the addition of a substance, by heating or cooling.

18. Coction

The cooking or heating of a substance at a moderate heat for an extended period.

19. Colliquation

The conjuction or melting together of two fusible substances.

20. Coloration

Tinging a substance by adding a dye or coloured tincture. Colouring can by either by tinging the whole body or by producing a surface coating.

21. Combustion

The burning of a sustance in the open air.

22. Comminution

The reduction of a substance into a powder, either by grinding, pulverising, or forcing it through a sieve.

23. Composition

The joining together of two different substances.

24. Conception

The marriage or union of the male and female aspects of substances.

25. Concoction

The cooking or heating of a mixture of substances at a moderate heat for an extended period.

26. Congelation

The conversion of a thin flowing liquid into a congealed thick substance, often by heating.

27. Conglutination

The conversion of a substance into a gluey mass, often by a putrefaction.

28. Conjunction

The joining of two opposite components, often seen as the union of the male and female, the subtle and gross, or even the elements.

29. Contrition

The reduction of a substance into powder only by means of fire.

30. Copulation

A conjunction, or joining of two opposite components, seen through the metaphor of the union of the male and female, or the union of the fixed and the volatile.

31. Corrosion

The eating up of a substance by an acid, alkali or corrosive material.

32. Cribation

The reduction of a substance to a powder by forcing through a sieve or mesh.

33. Crystallization

The formation of crystals out of a solution of the substance usually in water, either by their gradual formation from the liquid, or by evaporation of the liquid.

34. Dealbation

The making of the black substance of the alchemical process become brilliant white.

35. Decantation

It is aprocess of pouring gently and slowly a liquid (or Solution) conatined in a vessel, out of a mixture of the said liquid and other insoluble solid substnces, without disturbing those solid substances,which are deposited at the bottom as sediment.

36. Decoction

The digestion of a substance in the flask without the addition of any other material.

37. Decrepitation

The crackling and spliiting apart of substances, for example common salt, on heating.

38. Deliquium

The reduction of a solid placed in a damp place to a liquid by its absorbing water from the air.

39. Descension

When the subtle or active part of a substance is made to go down to the bottom of a flask, rather than ascend as a vapour.

40. Dessication

The drying or removal of all the moisture in a substance.

41. Detonation

The explosive burning of substances on heating, for example substances mixed with nitre.

42. Digestion

The slow modification of a substance by means of a gentle heat.

43. Disintegration

The breaking down or dissociation of a substance into different parts.

44. Dissociation

The breaking down or disintegration of a substance into different parts.

45. Dissolution

The dissolving or transforming of a substance into a liquid.

46. Distillation

The separation of a volatile component from a substance by heating so as to drive off the component as a vapour which is condensed and collected in a cooler part of the apparatus.

47. Dilution

It is method of mixing one liquid with another liquid. The more one liquid is added, the more weak the other liquid becomes in strength.

48. Drug

A substance which alter the function or nutrition of a part of the body. It has the capacity to effect a change in the human or animals in health or disease.

49. Ebullition

An effervescence produced through fermentation.

50. Edulceration

The washing of a salty substance till all the salts are removed.

51. Elaboration

The general term for the process of separating the pure from the impure, and leading a sustance towards perfection, which can be done through a variety of means and processes.

52. Elevation

The raising of the subtle parts of a substance upwards, away from the bodily residues, into the upper parts of the vessel.

53. Elixeration

The conversion of a substance into an elixir.

54. Evaporation

The removal of the watery part of a substance by gentle heating, or being left a long time in a dry place.

55. Exaltation

An operation by which a substance is raised into a purer and more perfect nature.

56. Exhalation

The release of a gas or air from a substance.

57. Extraction

The preparation of the subtler and purer parts of a substance, usually by macerating it in alcohol. The extract can then be separated from the residue.

58. Fermentation

The rotting of a substance, usually of an organic nature, often accompanied by the release of gas bubbles.

59. Filtration

The process or removing the grosser parts of a substance by passing through a strainer, filter or cloth.

60. Fixation

The make a volatile subject fixed or solid, so that it remains permanently unaffected by fire.

61. Fulmination

The preparation of a fulminate or explosively unstable form of a metal. Sometimes applied to any process in which a sudden eruptive event occurs.

62. Fumigation

The alteration of a substance by exposing it to a corroding smoke.

63. Fusion

The joining of powdered substances together, or the conversion of a substance into a new form, by means of an extremely high degree of heat, sometimes using a flux.

64. Glutination

Turning a substance into a gluey, glutinous mass.

65. Gradation

The gradual purification of a substance, often through a series of stages.

66. Granulation

The reduction of a substance to grains or powder. There are various means of doing this - pounding, grinding, using thermal shock by heating and rapid cooling, and many others.

67. Grinding

The reduction of substances to a powder, usually through the use of a mortar and pestle.

68. Humectation

A process by which humidity is given to the substance, usually not by the direct additon of liquid, but by a gradual process of absorbing moisture.

69. Ignition

The self-calcination of a substance by it burning itself in a crucible.

70. Imbibition

The feeding of a process by the gradual and continuing addition of some substance.

71. Impastation

When the matter undergoing putrefaction thickens or congeals into the consistency of molten black pitch.

72. Impregnation

The alchemical process is sometimes paralleled with the gestation of a child. Thus impregnation follows from the union or copulation of the male and female, and leads to the generation of a new substance.

73. Inceration

The making of a substance into a soft waxy consistency, usually by combining it with water.

74. Incineration

The conversion of a substance to ashes by means of a powerful fire.

75. Incorporation

The mingling of mixed bodies into a conglomerate mass.

76. Ingression

This occurs when substances combine in such a manner that they cannot afterwards be separated.

77. Inhumation

To bury under the earth, sometimes used to mean any process that buries the active substance in a dark earthy material. Also applied to placing a flask in the warm heat of a dung bath.

78. Liquefaction

The turning of a solid material into a liquid, either by melting or dissolving.

79. Lixiviation

The oxidation of sulphide ores by exposing them to air and water. This forms vitriols.

80. Luting

The sealing of a flask or other apparatus through the use of a lute, or resinous paste which once applied sets hard and produces an airtight seal.

81. Maturation

A general term applied to identify the appearance of a degree of perfection in the work.

82. Melting

The reduction of a metal or substance to a liquid through heating.

83. Mortification

Here the substance undergoes a kind of death, usually through a putrefaction, and seems to have been destroyed and its active power lost, but eventually is revived.

84. Multiplication

The operation by which the powder of projection has its power multiplied.

85. Precipitation

The descent of a substance out of a solution. The precipitate descends to the bottom of the flask.

86. Preparation

The process by which superfluous substances are removed from the matter and that which is wanting is added to it.

87. Projection

The throwing of a ferment or tincture onto a substance in order to effect a transformation of the substance.

88. Prolectation

The separation of a substance into a subtle and more coarse part by the thinning or rarefaction of the subtler parts of the substance, rather than the coarsening of the earthy part.

89. Pulverisation

The breaking down of a substance to smaller fragments through being repeatedly struck with a blunt instrument, such as a hammer, or mallet.

90. Purgation

The purging or purifying of a sustance by it casting forth a gross part.

91. Putrefaction

The rotting of a substance, often under a prolonged gentle moist heat. Usually the matter becomes black.

92. Quinta Essentia

The making of a quintessence, or highly elevated form of a substance.

93. Rarefaction

The making of a substance extremely subtle or thin and airy.

94. Rectification

The purification of the matter by means of repeated distillations, the distillate being again distilled.

95. Reiteration

The repetition of a process, particularly applied to circular distillation, in which the distillate is returned to the vessel, and the process continued for many cycles.

96. Resolution

This occurs when substances which are mixed together become violently separated by being placed into a solution. Thus milk is in this sense resolved by vinegar. This process is similar to coagulation.

97. Restinction

Here a substance at white heat is brought to perfection by being quenched in an exalting liquid.

98. Reverberation

An ignition or calcination at a high temperature, in a reverberating furnace.

99. Revivification

The bringing of a mortified matter back to life, or reactivating it.

100. Rubification

The making of the matter in the alchemical process from white to red.

101. Segregation

The separation of a composite substance into its parts.

102. Separation

The making of two opposite components separate from each other. Often alternated with the conjunction process.

103. Stratification

An operation which produces layers in the substance in the flask.

104. Subduction

The separation of abstraction downward of the subtle part, as in filtration.

105. Sublimation

This occurs when a solid is heated and gives off a vapour which condenses on the cool upper parts of the vessel as a solid, not going through a liquid phase. An example is sal ammoniac.

106. Subtilation

The separation of the subtle part of a substance from the gross.

107. Transudation

This occurs if the essence appears to sweat out in drops during a descending distillation.

108. Trituration

The reduction of a substance to a powder, not necessarily by the use of grinding, but by the application of heat.

109. Vitrification

The making of a substance into a glass but strong heating and sometimes the addition of lime.

110. Vitriolification

The making of a vitriol. Most often from a metal by the direct action of oil of vitriol, but sometimes by a more indirect route.

Appendix 2

Prescription Writing

Prescription means the selection of the remedy which the physician thinks to be the most appropriate for his patient, if the physician serves the required medicine from his own stock, no question of writing a prescription arises. Only recording of the medicine, potency and the circumstances under which the medicine was prescribed may be done in his diary (case diary) for future reference. But if he desires to get his prescription served, he should give directions in such a manner as to cause no difficulty on the part of a compounder to dispense with it. The whole body of the prescription is conveniently divided into four parts.

1. **Superscription:** Consists in the letter R which is the relic of the days of astrology. It originally designated the symbol of the planet Jupiter. Now it stands for a Latin word recipe means to take.

2. **Inscription:** Contains the name of the remedy, which is to be taken by the patient, its potency, its quantity and the vehicle.

3. **Subscription:** It means the direction or instructions to the compounder-how to dispense.

4. **Signature:** Gives directions to the patient how to take the medicine, together with prescriber's signature and registration number with date.

Abbreviations, notations, etc., used in prescription writing:

Aa	= Ana	= of each
Aq. dest.	= Aqua destillata	= distilled water before antecibum meals
Ad	= Ad libitum.	= To the desired amount, at pleasure; freely
Aq bull	= Aqua bulliens	= boiling water
Aq comm	= Aqua communis	= common water
Ad us exter	= Ad usumexternum	= for external use
Agit, a, us	= Agita ante	= Shake before using
Aur	= usum	= Thc ear or ears
Alt noc	= Alternis nocta	= every other night
B.D.	= Bis in die	= Twice daily
B.I.D.	= Bis in die	= Twice in a day
bol	= bolus	= a large pull
Bib	= Bibe	= drink B.P. = Boiling point
C	= Cim	= with
C	= Centum	= A hundred = Dubuc centerneter
cc	= Capitat	= Let him take
Cap	= Capiat	
Cib	= Cibus	= Food or meal
Cito disp	= Cito despern setur	= Let it be
dispensed c.m.	= Cras mane	= Let it be dispensed quickly
c.n.	= Cras nocte	= Tomorrow night

c.v.	= Cras Vespere	= Tomorrow evening
Coch	= Cochlears	= Spoon
Coach, amp-	= Coachleare ampum	= Spoonful, by spoonful
Coch mag.	= Cochleare magnum	= Large spoonful
Coch med	= Cochleare parvum	= A teaspoonful
Comp	= Compositus	= Compound
Confricamen	= Confricamentum	= A liniment
Cuj	= Cujus	= Of which
Cyath	= Cyathus	= Cup, wine-glass
D.	= Dosis	= Dose
d.	= da	= Give (thou)
dec	= decanote	= Pour off
decimus	= decimus	= the tenth
det	= detur	= Give
Dieb alt	= Diebas alternis	= on alternative days
dil	= dilute	= dilute, diluted
dim	= dimidus	=one half
Div	= Divide	= make into parts
Din P	= Divide in	=Let it be divided into equal parts
De, d, in d	= De cie in diem	= from day to day
d.r.d.	= dinur tables doses	= gives of such doses
ft. H.	= Fiait Haustus	= make a draught
ft mist.	= Fait misture	= make a mixture
Ft.	= Fiat	= Let it be made, mak
ft. Pulv.	= Fiat Pulvis	= make a power
ft. Pil	= Fiat Pilula	= make a pill

ft Linim	= Fiat Linimetum	= let a liniment be made
ft Cerat	= Fait ceratum	= Let a cerate be made
garg	= Gargarisma	= gargle
gm	= gram	
gr	= gram	
Gt. Gtt.	= Gutta, Gurrac	= drops
H	= Hora	= an hour
H.S.	= Hora Somni	= at bed time
h.d.	= Hora decubitus	= at bed time
H.S.S.	= Hora somnidus	= to be taken at bed time sumen
Hor	= Horis	= hour
Habt	= Habeat	= let him have
In d	= In die	= in a day
lac	= lac	= milk
lin	= linimentum	= liniment
lat. dol	= lateri dolente	= to the painful side
M.	= Misce	= Mix
m	= minim	= a drop
Mitt. tal	= mitte tables	= Send such
mag	= magnum	= large
mist	= mistura mixture	
Mode Prace	= mode praescript	= as prescribed script
M.P.	= Melting point	
Mor. dict.	= Moro dicto	= To be used in the manner directed
N.O.	= Natural order	= Family

Specimens of Prescription Writing

Case No 1: for Arthritis deformans

Patient's Name : Mrs. Susmita Sen

Sex: Female Age: 39 years

Rx	i)	S1	3D	-5 ml
	ii)	C2	3D	-5 ml
	iii)	C11	3D	-5 ml
	iv)	F1	3D	-5 ml

Ft. mist. in aqua dest.

Zi-T.d. x 7 days.

v) G.E -15ml

p.a.a./q.i.d. x 7 days.

Report thereafter

Signature :
Date:
Regn. No.

Case No.2: for Acute dysentery

Patient's Name : Mr. B.B. Sinha

Sex: Male Age: 55 years

Rx	i)	Sl	3D	-5 ml
	ii)	S10	3D	-5 ml
	iii)	C13	3D	-5 ml
	iv)	A2	3D	-5 ml

Ft. Mist in aqua dest

Zi-after every 10 mins. till patient recovers. :

Signature :
Date :
Regn. No .

Appendix 3

Count Cesare Mattei (1809-1896)

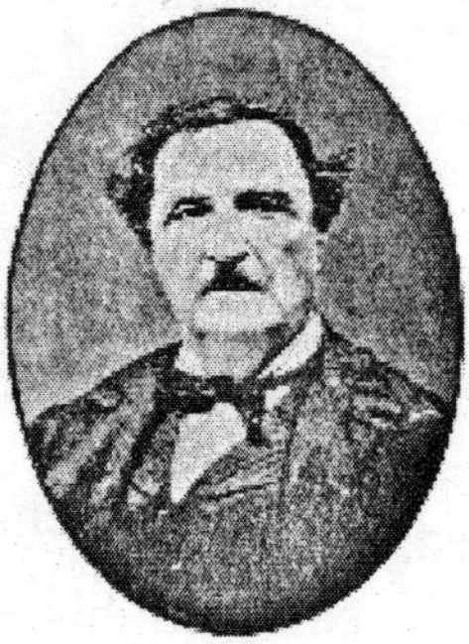

11.1.1809	born in Bologna
1850	Beginnings of the electrical Homoeopathy in the house of his parents
1860	Increasing interest in its work; also free treatment of without means
1867	Report over 156 healings of for patients incurably held first brochure over the new welfare procedure: "Brevi notizie sull Pmiopatia etc."
1869	Treatments with electrical Homoeopathie in the hospital pc. Theresa in Rome Attendance by Dr. Carl-Friedrich Zimpel and Dr. Arthur Lutze with Mattei
since 1870	Retreat on the Rocchetta, where it treated far patients (allegedly also duke Ludwig von Bayern and Czar Alexander II.)
1885-1896	Contact to Theodor Krauss
3.4.1896	Death

Theodor Krauss (1864-1924)

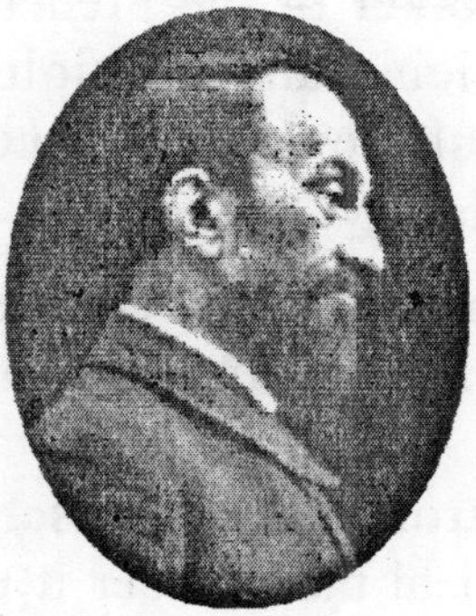

3.11.1864	born in Beraun (Boehmen)
until 1870	Youth years with his grandfather (Homoeopath and pupil of cock man)
1881	first contact with the electrical Homoeopathy
1883	Death of the grandfather and entrance into the Consortium for Electrical Homoeopathy, Regensburg
since 1883	Further learning of the Electro Homoeopathy
1885-1896	Contact to Count Cesare Mattei, the founder of the Electro Homoeopathy
Starting from 1885	Establishment of a committee for the spreading of the Electro Homoeopathy, constant scientific coworker of the Regensburger Consortiums, literary activity (and A. "sheets for Electrical Homoeopathy", "the electrical homoeopathy ABC"). Its works appeared finally in six different languages
1.10.1890	Scientific director/conductor of the Consortiums, shifted to Regensburg

for approx. 1890

Coworker of the French homoeopathischen physician and physiologist Dr. Encausse; Translation of Dr. Encausse's "synthetic physiology"

since 1896 Promotion of the electrical Homoeopathie in Germany, with lecture journeys, establishment of associations, training of elektrohomoeopathischen physicians and practical men (under it university courses in Berlin)

1900 Graduation

1909 Receipt of the title "professor for the chair of the okkulten and hermetic medicine" of the "Ecole supérieure libre" "ad honores" for a price work

Approx. 1917

Development of the JSO complex Heilweise in co-operation with the pharmacist Johannes Sonntag and the homoeopathischen physician Dr. med. Johannes of thing fields

31.3.1918 Assumption of the editorship of the "monthly magazine for compound Homoeopathie"

1.10.1924 Death

Dr. Carl Friedrich Zimpel (1801-1879)

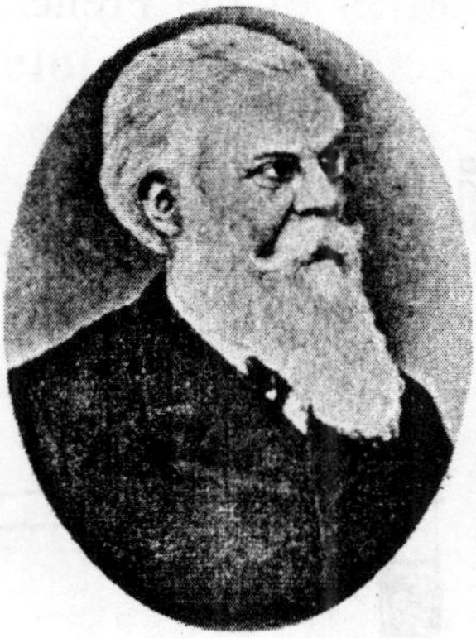

11.12.1801	Born in Sprottau, Lower Silesia.
26.6.1879	In Pozzuoli (Campania) Zimpel became an officer, in later years he worked for various Railway administrations and companies in Germany and also abroad and received American citizenship. He spoke and wrote the English and the French language.
1849	Zimpel received the doctorate in medicine, he relocated to Italy.
1866	Meeting with the Italian Count Cesare Mattei, whose products he replicated. The present method "Spag. Zimpel" registered in GHP/ USHP. From Zimpel about 40 books between 1828 and 1879 are provable, many of it in French.
26.6.1879	Died in a hotel in Pozzuoli (southern Italy).

Appendix 4

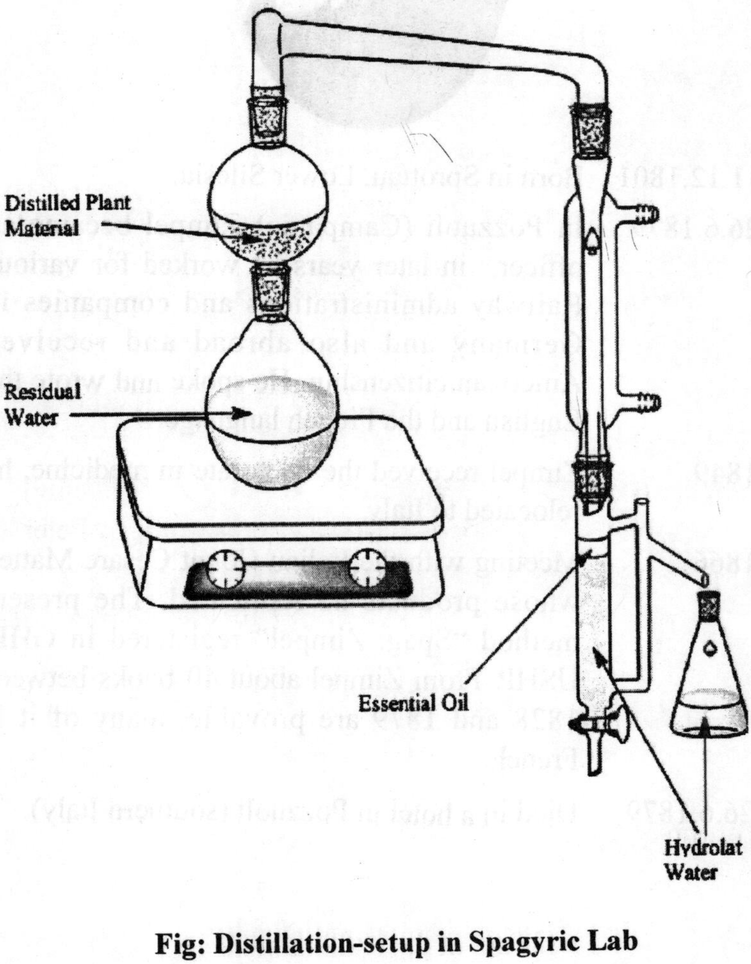

Fig: Distillation-setup in Spagyric Lab

Bibliography

1. Homoeopathic Pharmacopoeia of the U.S.A (American Institute of Homeopathy).
2. German Homoeopathic Pharmacopoeia (Medpharm Scientific Publishers, GmbH).
3. Alchemy by John Reid (Russell House, Illinois).
4. Die Grundgesetze der JSO-komplex-heilweise by Theodor Krauss (Sonntag J.Verlag).
5. Spagirisch heilen by Herta Richter and Michael Schunemann (Foitzick Verlag).
6. Alchemei der Neuzeit by Axel Helmstadter, (Wissenschaftliche Verlagsgesellschaft).
7. Pharmacodynamics in Electro Homeopathy by Dr.Debasish Kundu (B Jain Publishers).
8. Materia Medica and Practice of Medicine in Electro Homoeopathy by Dr. Debasish Kundu (Originals).
9. Pharmacodynamics in Spagyric Medicine (Plant Alchemy) by Dr. Debasish & Sudeshna Kundu, Forewored by Peter Morrell (Orignals).
10. Natural Medicines by Dr. Debasish Kundu & Dr. Malik A.K.Awan, Foreworded by Dr. Rui Oliviera (Kruger Brentt, U.K.).
11. Notes on Spagyrics by Dr. Debasish Kundu (Originals).
12. A Treatise on Spagyric Homoeopathic Pharmacy By Prof. Dr. Debasish Kundu Edited By Dr. Vijai Kant Agnihotri, Scientist, CSIR, Govt of India, Foreworded By Raffaele Pezzani, University of Padova, Italy (Originals).

Notes on Spagyrics

By Dr. Debasish Kundu

Rs. 395/- US $ 21.50 Paperback

In this book author briefly discusses the principles of Alchemy with some exceptional notes on Sexual and Spiritual Alchemy.

CONTENTS: Note to the Readers, Foreword, Preface, Introduction, History of Alchemy, Spagyrics, Principles of Spagyrics, The Quest for the Quintessence, Plant Alchemy, Energetic Spagyrics, The Three Philosophical Principles, Spagyric Electro-Homoeopathy, Energy in the Organism, Herbal Medicine, Spiritual Alchemy, Sexual Alchemy, Spagyric Meditation, Hermetic Philosophy, Fermentation and Distillation of Wine Spirit, Spagyric Experiments, Explanation of Some Spagyrics Terms, Bibliography

Materia Medica and Practice of Medicine in Electro-Homoeopathy

By Dr.Debasish Kundu

Rs. 395/- US $ 21.50 Paperback

CONTENTS: Foreword, Preface, Electrohomoeopathy-An Introduction, Life History of Count Cesare Mattei, Preparation of Electro Homoeopathic Remedies, Electrohomoeopathy Formulas, Constitution and Temperament, Materia Medica of Electrohomoeopathy Medicines, Examination of the Patient, General Rules for Using the Medicines, Practice of Medicine, Points for External Application, Chief Points and their Uses, Clinical Index, Bibliography

Treatise on Spagyric Homoeopathic Pharmacy

By Dr. Debasish Kundu & Dr. Vijay Kant Agnihotri, Sr. Scientist, CSIR, Foreworded By Prof. Raffaele Pezzani, University of Padova, Italy

Rs. 395/- US $ 21.50 Paperback

It features all necessary information about the method of preparations and formulations of Zimpel, Krauss and Bernus. It is the only book which has incorporated Spagyrics formulas of Zimpel brought back from the lost fragments of time.

According to Prof. Pezzani, it is definitely a valuable guide, a friend that every Electrohomeopathy (according to Mattei) practitioner should possess. It is a must have collection for everyone.

CONTENTS: Dedication, Foreword, Preface, Spagyric Homeopathic Pharmacy, Electrohomoeopathy Formulas, Spagyrics after Zimpel, Krauss and Bernus, Medicinal Plants, Tables of Essential Oil Yielding Plants, Bibliography

Materia Medica for the New Age Man

By Dr. Debasish Kundu, Dr A.Jayasuriya, Chancellor, The Open International University, Colombo and Edited by Dr. M Ahmed, Member, Bangladesh Homeopathy Board, Dhaka

Rs. 450/- US $ 24.50 Hardbound

This is the only book which covered all therapeutic schools of Homeopathy, from Gemmotherapy, Lithotherapy, Bach flower to Spagyric Homeopathy.

CONTENTS: Foreword to the Second Edition, Introduction, Introduction to Homeopathy, Evolution of Disease, Introduction to Vital Force, Miasms, Homeopathic Pharmacy, Case Taking, Doctrine of Dosage, Therapeutic Schools of Homeotherapeutics at a Glance, Nosodes and Sarcodes, Materia Medica, Clinical Index of Homeopathic Remedies, Mother Tinctures (External Use), Do's and Don'ts for Patients, Clinical Tips for Dummies, General Index of Remedies, References

Treatise on Electro-Homoeopathic Pharmacy

By Dr. Debasish Kundu & Dr.Ajit Singh, Forewórded By Prof. Fabio R Ambrosi, Chairman, Mattei Archieves, Italy

Rs. 195/- US $ 15.50 Paperback

CONTENTS: Foreword, Preface, Introduction to Electro Homoeopathic Pharmacy, Laboratory Equipments Used in Electro Homoeopathy Pharmacy, Vehicles used in Electrohomoeopathy, Sources of Electro Homoeopthic Medicines, Collection of Medicinal Plants, Cohobation: An Extraordinary Pharmacy, Methods of Preparation of Spagyric Medicines, Quality Control Procedures, Pharmacodynamics of Electrohomoeopathy Essences, Dosages and Mode of Administration, List of Medicinal Plants Used in

Electrohomoeopathic Remedies, Appendix 1: Terminology, Appendix 2: Prescription Writing, Appendix 3: Biographies, Appendix 4: Apparatus, Bibliography

Essentials of Acupuncture

By Dr. Debasish Kundu & Prof. Choo Led Sin, Chairman, International Federation of Acupuncture, Singapore

Rs. 995/- US $ 40.00 Hardbound

The Only Book which deals with Acupuncture Anaesthesia

CONTENTS: Preface, Introduction, History of Acupuncture, Philosophy of Acupuncture, Five Elements Theory, Diagnosis in Traditional Chinese Medicine, Evaluation and Diagnosis, The Concept of Qi, Management & Research on Some Disorders, How Acupuncture Works, Acupuncture Anesthesia, Laser Acupuncture, Auriculotherapy, Atlas of Acupuncture Points, Therapeutics of Common Ailments, Therapeutics of Common Ailments, Infertility, Impotence and Acupuncture, Acupuncture in Hairfall, Does Acupuncture Hurts, Related Therapies, Explanation of Some Terms, Marmapuncture, Bibliography

Cesare Mattei's Principles of Electro Homeopathy

Interpreted & Revised By Dr. Debasish Kundu

Rs. 395/- US $ 21.50 Paperback

The classic text has been Rewritten in simple language with much needed Interpretation & Revision. In some places the original French edition has been consulted, also enriched with footnotes wherever necessary.

CONTENTS: Preface by Editor, What is Electro-Homeopathy?, Names of the Electro-Homeopathic Remedies, General Information about the Electro-Homeopathic Remedies, Sphere of Action of the Remedies in Globules, General Remarks on the Electric Liquids, Their Mode of Application, Results of Experience, Doses and Method of Administration of the Remedies in Globules, Of Diagnosis, Principles and Rules for the Selection of the Appropriate Remedy, Easy Experiments for Beginners, Catalogue of Diseases Cured by Electro-Homeopathy, Appendix

Stepping Stones to Electo-Homoeopathy (Count Mattei's System of Medicine)

By A J L Gliddon(Original Edition with Vitiation of Blood and Lymph Theory)

Rs. 395/- US $ 21.50 Paperback

A brief insight into the discovery of electro homeopathy together with a rational explanation of the principles involved and the proposed medicines.

CONTENTS: Introduction , The Human Body, Count Mattei's Theories, Symptoms of Disease, The Electro-Homceopathic Remedies, The Globule Remedies, The Electricities, External Use of Electricities, External Use of Globules, Baths, Compresses, etc., How to Select the Remedies, How to Determine the Dose, Dilutions, Dry Globules, Table of Doses, Minute Doses, Effects of the Remedies, Other Hygienic Helps, Diet, Dress, Pure Air, etc.

Essentials of Trace Elements & Biochemic Medicine

By Prof. Dr. Debasish Kundu, Edited By Prof. Seyed Farzin Hassanzadeh Salehian Ph.D. (Iran)

Rs. 350/- US $ 19.00 Paperback

Cell Salts or Bioplasgens have always been considered an important part of healing in Homeopathy and Spagyrics. This book contains all essential materials concerning Trace Elements & Bioplasgen and their relationship with Spagyrics, Clinical Materia Medica with useful suggestions.

CONTENTS: Preface, Introduction to Trace Elements & Bioplasgens, The Functions of The Cell, Astrology and Bioplasgens, Minerals, Trace Elements, Materia Medica of the Bioplasgens, Bio-combinations, Bibliography

A Textbook on Food, Nutrition and Dietetics

By Dr. Debasish Kundu Editor Dr. Malik A.K. Awan Ph.D. (London), Associate Editor Prof. Seyed Farzin Hassanzadeh Salehian Ph.D.(Iran)

Rs. 495/- US $ 20.00 Paperback

CONTENTS: Preface, Relationship between Food, Nutrition & Health, History of Nutrition, Functions of Food, Digestion of Food, Food and Nutrition, Nutrition, Diet & Development, Nutrition & Diet Therapy, Nutrition for Infants, Children, Adults, Women and Elderly, Ideal Diet Plan, The Food Pyramid, Therapeutic Diet, Bibliography

Notes on MJT (Forensic Medicine & Toxicology)

By Dr. Debasish Kundu Ph.D. Assisted By Dr. Ravi Justin Raj NMD, LLB Edited By Dr. Malik A.K. Awan B.S., M.S. (Psychology), D.C.L., D.D. (U.S.A.), Ph.D. (London)

Rs. 550/- US $ 22.00 Paperback

CONTENTS: Part I: Forensic Medicine: Dedication , Preface , Introduction, Scope of Forensic Medicine, Aspects of Identification, Medico-legal Aspects of Death, Investigation of Death, Death by Asphyxia, Medico-legal Aspects of Injuries, Investigation of Wounds, Medico-legal Aspects of Sex Crimes, Medico-legal Aspects of Abortion, Forensic Pathology, Forensic Entomology, Radiation Poisoning, Medico-legal Sections in IPC, Cr PC, AND IE A, Part II: Toxicology: Introduction to Toxicology, General Approach to a Victim of Poison, Clinical Toxicology Laboratory, Practical Aspects of Analytical Toxicology, Toxicants of Public Health Hazard, Medical Toxicants, Environmental Toxicants, Abuse of Drugs, Natural Toxicants, Annexure I: Preparations of Reagents, Annexure II: Apparatuses, Annexure III: Glossary of Terms Used, Annexure IV: Abbreviations Used, Bibliography

Notes on Minor Surgery

By Dr. Debasish Kundu Ph.D. Guided & Edited by Dr. A.K. Banerjee M.B.B.S., M.D. (U.S.A.)

Rs. 395/- US $ 21.50 Paperback

CONTENTS: Part-I: Preface, Acharya Sushruta, Basic Surgical Procedures, Surgery of Some Common Conditions, Part II: Sterilisation, Suture Materials, Nomenclature of Operations, Planning for Operation, Anaesthesia,Operative Surgery, Postoperative Complications, Abscess Drainage, Venesection (Cut Down), Skin Grafting, Circumcision, Vasectomy, Hyderocele, Inguinal Hernia, Strangulated Inguinal Hernia, Femoral Hernia, Umbilical Hernia, Appendicetomy,

Abdominal Incisions, Peptic Ulcer, Vagotomy, Gastrojejumnostomy, Partial Gastrectomy, Closure of Perforated Peptic Ulcer, Right Hemicolectomy, Colostomy, Cholecystectomy, Choledocholithotomy (Supraduodenal), Spleenectomy, Lumbar Sympathectomy, Haemorrhoidectomy, Suprapubic Cystostomy, Prostatectomy, Exposure of Kidney , Exposure of the Ureter and Ureterolithotomy, Mastectomy, Thyroidectomy, Tracheostomy, Empyema Thoracis, Amputations, Bibliography

Principles and Practice of Naturopathy

By Dr. Debasish Kundu Editor Dr. Malik A. K. Awan Ph.D. (London) Associate Editor Prof. Sayed Farzin Hassanzadeh Salehian Ph.D.(Iran)

Rs. 750/- US $ 30.00 Paperback

CONTENTS: Foreword, Preface to the First Edition, Preface to the Third Edition, Naturopathy: Its Principles & Pioneers, Physiology, Food and Nutrition, Hygiene and Sanitation, Biology, Herbology, Medicinal Plants, Magnet Therapy, Yoga and Meditation, Massage Therapy, Medical Gymnastics, Chemistry, Bacteriology, Toxicology, Pathology, Osteology, Neurology, Ethics, Hydro Therapy and Helio Therapy, Colour Therapy, Fasting and Diet, Mud Therapy and Fango Therapy, Acupressure, Aromatherapy, Reflexology, Iridology, Vitamins and Balanced Diets, Bibliography

Diseases of Women (Adopted from Margaret Seifert's Krankheiten Der Franen)

By Dr. Shefalika Kundu, Edited By Dr. Debasish Kundu & Dr. Sudeshna Kundu

Rs. 350/- US $ 19.00 Paperback

The book is intended as a handbook on diseases of women with their Electrohomeopathic treatment. Besides an update on the literature on Contraception using Spagyrics , entirely new topics Anatomy of Uterus and Stages of development in Pregnancy are added.

CONTENTS: Preface to the Second Edition, Foreword to the First Edition, Preface, Introduction, Anatomy and Physiology of Sexual Organs of Women, General View of Treatment, Diseases and Their Treatment, Hygienic Care of the Body and Toilet, Anatomy of Uterus in Pregnancy, Notes on Various Diseases, Family Planning, Contraception in Electrohomoeopathy,Diet, Index of Diseases Discussed, Bibliography

Lectures on Materia Medica & Therapeutics

By Dr. H. D. Banerjee, Foreworded By M V Mattei, Thoroughly Revised & Edited By Prof. Dr. Debasish Kundu

Rs. 225/- US $ 18.00 Paperback

CONTENTS: Preface to the Third Edition, Preface to the Second Edition, Foreword to the First Edition, Introduction, On Electro-Homoeopathic Principles, On Principles of Orthodox School, On Homeopathic Principles , On Objections to Electro-Homoeopathy, Chemical Analysis of the Remedies, Dynamisation of the Remedies, On Minute Doses, On Frequency of the Doses, Purgatives in Electro-Homoeopathy, On Prescription Writing, Materia Medica & Therapeutics, On Therapeutics of the Remedies

Principles & Art of Cure in Electrohomeopathy

By Prof. Dr.Debasish Kundu Ph.D.

Rs. 195/- US $ 15.00 Paperback

CONTENTS: Introduction to Electrohomeopathy, Philosophy, The Discoverer, Principles of Nature, Introduction to Electrohomeopathy Medicines, The Iris science, Sources and preparation of Electrohomeopathy Medicines, Cohobation, Spagyric Tinctures, Classification of Electrohomeopathy Medicines, Classification, Preparation and Therapeutics uses of Electrohomeopathy Medicines, Potentisation of Electrohomeopathy Medicines and Electric fluids, Preparation and Therapeutic uses of Ointments and Lotions, Points for application Electric Fluids, Ointments and Lotions, Plain talks on using the medicines, Potentisation and Bio-Magnetism, The Similia of Electrohomeopathy, The Scientific basis of Electrohomeopathy System of Medicine, World's present day need of Electrohomeopathy, Clinical Index.

A Clinical Treatise on Cancer

By Prof. Dr.Debasish Kundu Ph.D. Foreworded By Dr. B.B. Upreti, Ph. D. General Secretary, All Nepal Electro-Homeo Medical Association, Hetauda, Nepal

Rs. 195/- US $ 15.00 Paperback

CONTENTS: Introduction, The Increase of Cancer and it's Causes, The Treatment of Cancer, Diet for Patients, Hygienic Care of the Patients

Books Published By LBO Publishing, 700 N Valley St., Suite B PMB 11884 Anaheim, CA 92801, USA Marketed In India Exclusively By Originals, Delhi

Pharmacodynamics in Spagyric Medicine(Plant Alchemy)

By Dr. Debasish Kundu & Dr.Sudeshna Kundu, Edited by Gisela Bruckel(Germany), El Akrem Hayouni (Tunisia), Forwarded by Dr.Peter Morrell (U.K.), Prof. Luigi Vernacchia & Dr.Fabio Ambrosi (Italy) Printed on Art Paper, USD ($) 70.00, Hardbound

It is the only trusted book to learn Sacred Alchemical Philosophy with Practical Laboratory Spagyrics, it covers from history & principles of Alchemy to the rarest topic Botanical Consciousness in Spagyrics, besides, Alchemy and the Zodiac Connection and how Spagyric Medicines work. In addition, detailed Pharmaceutical Process which are being carried out in most modern laboratories : from Apparatus, Vehicles, Sources of Medicines, Preparation of Spagyric Essences, quality control like Phytochemical Analysis, etc. , all major Spagyric Methods known to mankind, incl., Mattei, Zimpel, Junius, Solaris, Krauss,etc., besides the sacred Indian, Arabian and Chinese methods, Doctrine of Dosage, and much more. An Encyclopedia of Spagyrics or Plant Alchemy in one nutshell.

This work is edited by Gisela Bruckel, who is a Pharmacist and her Pharmacy in Wurzburg was the Main Dealer of Mattei Remedies in Europe till M V Mattei era, and Prof. El Akrem Hayouni, World famous authority on Plant Alchemy.

CONTENTS: Foreword, Preface, Part 1: Introduction to Spagyric Medicine, History of Alchemy, Principles of Spagyrics, The Simila of Alchemy, Difference Between Homoeopathy and Spagyric Homoeopathy, Botanical Consciousness in Spagyrics, Micronutrients and Spagyrics, Alchemy and the Zodiac Connection, How Spagyric Medicines Work, Alchemy and Spagyrics, Spagyrics : The Future in Medicine, Part 2: Pharmacy in Plant Alchemy, Pharmaceutical Process, Laboratory Apparatus, Vehicles Used in Plant Alchemy, Sources of Medicines, Preparation of Spagyric Essence, Spagyric Essence by Cohobation Method, Phytochemical Analysis of Plants, Different Spagyric Methods, Quality Control Procedures, Safety Measures in Laboratory, Doctrine of Dosage, Medicinal Plants, Terminology, Appendix, Bibliography

Mysticism, Romance & Secrets of Count Cesare Mattei (With Properly Transcripted Secret Formulas)

By Prof. Dr. Debasish Kundu , Ph.D. (U.S.A.)

Printed on Art Paper, USD ($) 40.00 Hard Bound

It is the Bible of Mattei Electrohomoeopathy : covering the true life of Cesare Mattei and properly transcripted Empirical Formulas & Secret Pharmacy of Electrohomoeopathy, incl. Medicinal Plants Used by Cesare Mattei.

Contributors-Prof. Raffaele Pezzani, University of Padova, Italy, Dr. Fabio R. Ambrosi, University of Sapienza, Rome, Italy, Prof. El Akrem Hayouni, University of Manouba, Tunisia, Allesandro Rapparini, Vice Pres., Archivio Museo Cesare Mattei, Bologna, Italy, Prof. Peter Morrell, Formerly Honorary Research Associate, History of Medicine, Staffordshire University, U.K., Dr. Terry Mitchell, Alchemist & Director, Phylak GmbH, U.K., Willow Morningsky, Spagyrist & Psychologist, Southern Oregon University, Ashland, Oregon, U.S.A. etc.

CONTENTS: Introduction, Dedication, Note to the Readers, Acknowledgements, Alchemist's Prayer, Preface, The Castle of Love, The Mystery Unveiled, Emerald Tablet of Cesare Mattei, Mysticism & Romance of Cesare Mattei, Electro Homoeopathy Pharmacology, Medicinal Plants Used by Cesare Mattei, Glossary of Pharmacological Terms, Bibliography

For Further Information and Ordering:
Originals/Low Price Publications
A-6, Second Floor, Nimri Commercial Centre,
Ashok Vihar Phase-4, Delhi - 110 052 (India)
Tel.: +91 11 2730 2453 Fax: 011 4706 1936
Mobile: 98100-12366
Website: www.Lppindia.com,
e-mail: info@Lppindia.com
info@Lbopub.com